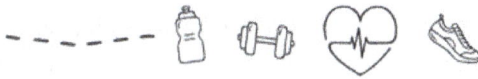

LOVE YOUR BODY

Unlock the Secrets to Reinvent Your Life, Change Your Body, and Improve Your Mind

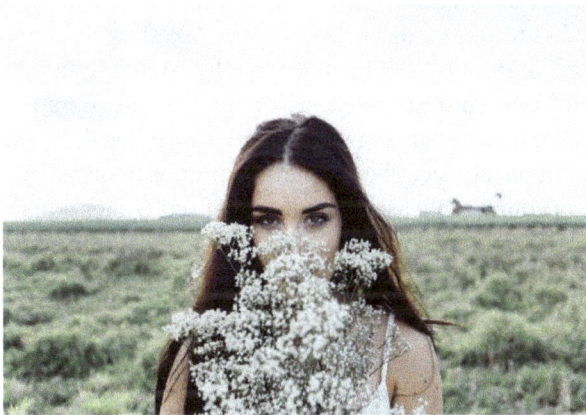

Dr. Gillian Keys Pomroy,
Dr. Anna Bernardi

THANK YOU FOR
PURCHASING THIS BOOK!

Table of Contents

LOVE YOUR BODY

Introduction: Your Beginner's Guide to a Better Life.......1

Chapter 1: Clean Eating 3

Chapter 2: Finding Physical and Mental Energy 13

Chapter 3: Getting Started............................... 22

Chapter 4: The Dos and Don'ts of Loving Your Body 28

Chapter 5: Shopping and Cooking..................................35

Chapter 6: Believe in Yourself to Reach Your Goals 46

Chapter 7: A Day in the Life of Self-love 53

Conclusion It's Time to Start Changing Your Life! 59

Bibliography.. 60

INTERMITTENT DIET FOR WOMEN OVER 50

Introduction... 65

Chapter 1: Introduction to the Intermittent Fasting
Diet.. 66

Chapter 2: Types of Intermittent Fasting...................... 69

Chapter 3: The Benefits of Fasting for Women Over 50.77

Chapter 4: Balancing Hormones and Boosting Energy . 82

Chapter 5: Definitive Weight Loss and Increased
Mental Clarity 88

Chapter 6: What You Need to Know 96

Chapter 8: Maintaining Your Weight..........................150

Chapter 9: Intermittent Fasting Foods 154

Chapter 10: Changing Your Habits and Your Mindset
to Change Your Body 162

Conclusion 185

References...187

KETO DIET OVER 50

Introduction...193

Chapter 1: The History of the Ketogenic Diet: What is
Keto? 196

Chapter 2: Types of Ketogenic: SKD, TKD, and CKD .. 205

Chapter 3: Why Women Over 50?..............................213

Chapter 4: Balance Hormones and Boost Energy.........221

Chapter 5: Definitive Weight Loss and Increased
Mental Clarity 229

Chapter 6: After Diet Appetite Control 243

Chapter 7: Food for Stable Blood Sugar Levels........... 252

Chapter 8: Changing Your Habits and Your Mindset
to Change Your Body 259

Chapter 9: Reaching Your Goal 267

Chapter 10: Charged with Optimism...........................275

Conclusion 282

References... 285

Introduction: Your Beginner's Guide to a Better Life

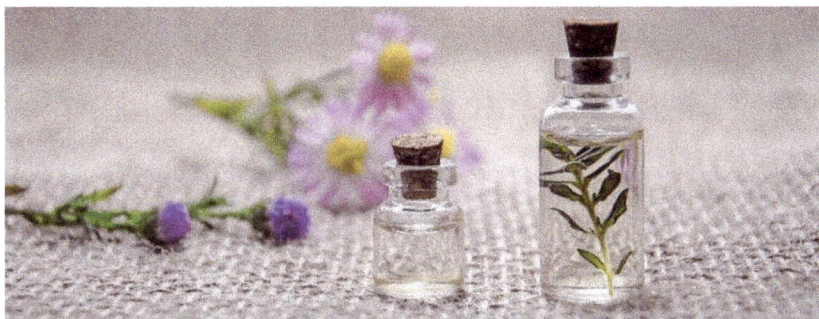

We all wish for a better life. But the question is, how do you achieve it?

The best way to do this is to start working towards the life you dream of having. The fact is, nothing will happen if you just sit there dreaming of what could be but not really do anything about it. There's no time like the present to start loving yourself more and working hard to improve yourself from within.

The good news is that you're reading this book right now and it's the perfect guide to help motivate you to love the body you're in. This book also aims to encourage further improvement by following a healthy diet and learning how to take care of yourself. If you want your life to become better, you need to start with yourself. Unless you feel happy, motivated, and confident in yourself, you might find it extremely challenging to go for the other things you truly want to achieve.

In this book, you'll learn all about how you can start improving your life by starting with yourself. With that being said, let's begin!

Chapter 1:
Clean Eating

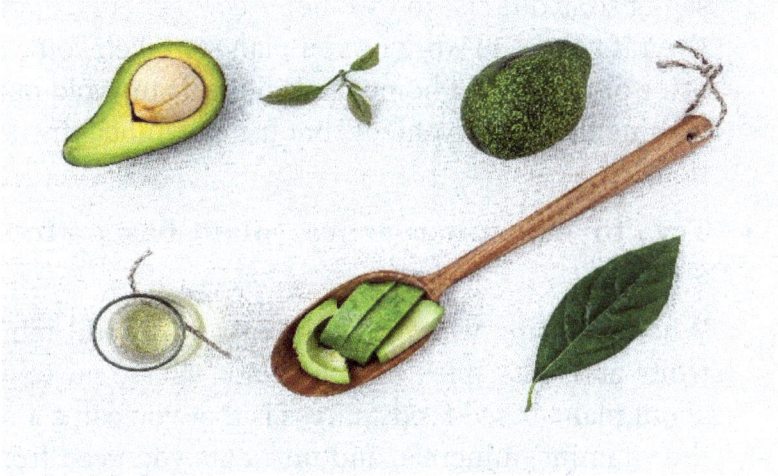

Essentially, clean eating is a diet—a specific way of eating. But you can also see it as a kind of lifestyle which helps improve your overall health and well-being. Simple as this diet is, clean eating involves a couple of key principles. These principles align with the basic principles of any healthy diet:

- **Choose real foods**

  This is the most common basic principle of healthy eating. If you want to start clean eating, then you must try to avoid refined or processed foods. Instead, opt for real foods which you either eat raw or which you can use to create healthy and tasty dishes. Often, the reason people go for packaged foods is convenience. This may be okay sometimes, but you can still go for products which contain real foods without artificial ingredients.

- **Eat for the purpose of nourishment**

  It's important for you to eat balanced, healthy meals and snacks regularly. Make sure these are nourishing and you don't rush through your meals. If possible, eat home-cooked meals, whether you cook them yourself or someone else in your home cooks them for you. Even if you go to work or you plan to travel, you can bring along packed home-cooked meals to avoid purchasing those "convenient" but usually unhealthy options.

- **Try to consume more plant-based food sources**

  When choosing what foods to eat, try to add more fruits and vegetables on your plate. The great thing about plant-based food sources is that you can get all the vitamins, minerals, and nutrients you need from them. For instance, we all need protein, right? You don't just have to get your protein from meat. There are a lot of plant-based food sources which contain protein such as whole grains, lentils, peas, beans, and much more.

- **Limit or avoid meat as much as possible**

  More and more studies have shown that limiting or avoiding meat is beneficial for overall health. Although clean eating doesn't require you to become a vegan or vegetarian, cutting back on your meat consumption can improve your health. You may have meat on occasion, but it's best to make plant-based foods the staple in your diet.

- **Limit added sugar**

  Unfortunately, a lot of people eat foods which are high in added sugars and this is never a good thing. If you want to clean up your eating habits, you may want to limit those common sweet treats such as baked goods, candy, soda, and the like. You may also want to check the sugar content of any "health foods" you plan to buy as these may contain added sugars too. This is why it's better to go for whole foods because you won't have to worry about any hidden ingredients.

- **Cut back on sodium**

  Sugar isn't the only issue when it comes to the foods we eat. Most people consume far more sodium than we actually need. If you want to limit your sodium intake, avoiding processed foods is an important step because these products typically contain high amounts of sodium. Although you can use salt in clean eating recipes, make sure to use this ingredient sparingly. Add it to bring out the flavors of your foods, not as the main flavor of your food.

- **Clean up your lifestyle**

  Part of clean eating is also adopting a cleaner lifestyle. Aside from eating the right foods, you should also get enough physical activity or exercise, get enough sleep each night, and learn how to manage stress properly. Also, connect with the people in your life. Talk to them, laugh with them, take a walk with them, and more. All of these will help you become a happier, healthier, and cleaner person.

- **It's about the environment too**

  The more people start clean eating, the more our planet will benefit. If more of us consume plant-based sources, this can help reduce the demand of the animal agricultural industry which, unfortunately, has a lot of negative effects on the environment. So, you can think about it this way: clean eating doesn't just have a positive impact on your life, it also has a positive impact on the planet.

The Health Benefits of Following a Healthy, Well-Balanced Diet

Now that you know more about clean eating, let's focus on the benefits of following such a diet. Following a healthy, clean diet means that you eat a lot of colorful fruits and veggies along with lean proteins, whole grains, starches, and good fats. It also means that you avoid foods which contain high amounts of unhealthy fats, sugar, and salt. Clean eating is an excellent diet and lifestyle because it provides you with these health benefits:

- **Weight loss**

  This is one thing a lot of people seem to be struggling with and it also happens to be one of the main frustrations of people all over the world. Although you may follow different kinds of diets, you just can't seem to shed those unwanted pounds! This may be because you're not following the diet properly or the type of diet you're following isn't suitable for your body.

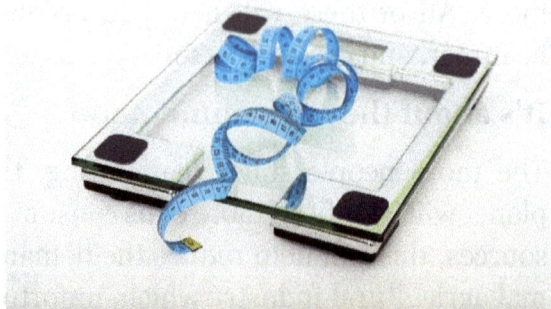

When you follow a healthy, well-balanced diet, it can help you reach your weight-loss goals. Aside from this, losing weight may also help in reducing the risk of developing chronic health conditions.

- **Reduced risk of developing cancer**

  Consuming too many processed and refined foods may lead to different types of health conditions which may increase your risk of developing certain cancers. But if you go for whole, healthy foods, this may help reduce the risk. In fact, there are a lot of fruits, vegetables, and plant-based food sources which can even help protect you against these life-threatening conditions.

- **It helps in the management of diabetes**

  Clean eating allows people who suffer from diabetes to manage their levels of blood glucose, maintain healthy levels of cholesterol and blood pressure, and delay or prevent the complications that usually accompany this condition.

- **It promotes the health of the heart**

  Heart disease is a very common condition all around the world. According to research, different kinds of heart disease can be avoided by making changes in your lifestyle, such as eating healthier foods and having enough exercise or physical activity. Clean eating is the perfect diet to promote the health of the heart. So, if you already have heart disease or you are at high risk of developing the condition, this diet can be very beneficial for you.

- **It strengthens the bones and teeth**

  This is another excellent benefit of clean eating. As you follow a healthy and balanced diet, you're able to get enough of the essential nutrients each day. Nutrients such as magnesium and calcium are commonly found in plants and are essential for the strength of our teeth and bones. These nutrients also help prevent the development of osteoarthritis and osteoporosis later in life.

- **It may improve your mood**

  Many recent studies are finding a close relationship between our mood and our diet. For instance, diets that have a high glycemic level may increase the risk of developing the symptoms of depression. But if you follow a diet composed mainly of whole foods, you won't have to worry about this. Also, the more your diet makes you feel strong and healthy, the happier you will become.

- **It helps maintain the health of the brain to improve cognitive functions**

  Eating healthy foods helps maintain the health of your brain. This is very important since the brain oversees all the processes and functions of your body. Clean eating may help prevent cognitive decline so you may want to consider it if you want your mind to function well as you grow older.

- **It promotes gut health**

  Our gut is host to an entire ecosystem of bacteria, some of which are good while others are bad. A healthy diet promotes the health of our gut since the foods you eat are also the foods which nourish the good bacteria. This helps strengthen your immune system in order to reduce the risk of developing different kinds of illnesses and diseases.

- **It helps you get a good night sleep each night**

    Following a healthy diet may also help you sleep better each night. Most of the time, our sleeping patterns get disrupted by certain factors, such as drinking alcohol, obesity, and an unhealthy diet. When you clean up your life by eliminating these, you will be able to get enough rest to keep you healthy and strong.

The Most Common Issues People Have with Food and How to Overcome Them

Although food is one of our basic needs, a lot of us struggle with it. In the past, people didn't have a lot of options, so they ate similar things. However, currently there are endless selections of fresh produce, whole foods, processed foods, refined foods, and more. So, it can be overwhelming to follow just one diet and keep things simple.

Apart from finding it a challenge to eat healthy foods as opposed to the scrumptious but unhealthy options we are so used to eating, some people also succumb to a number of common issues with food. The sad thing with these issues is that overcoming them can seem like an impossible task, especially when you don't know how to do this or where to start. If all this seems familiar to you, then you may be suffering from one type of food issue or another. To help you overcome whatever it is you're dealing with, let's look at these common issues and how to deal with them:

1. **Over-eating**

    When it comes to eating, or rather, when it's time to stop eating, a lot of people struggle with self-control.

Consuming too many calories each day or eating too much each meal or in a single sitting are very common habits which are very challenging to break. Unfortunately, overeating leads to weight gain which increases your risk of developing chronic diseases.

Also, overeating prevents you from reaching your fitness, wellness, and health goals. If you tend to overeat, you may find it difficult to start a clean eating lifestyle as well. If you want to overcome this, here are some tips which may help you:

- Avoid doing other things while you're eating so you can focus more on what you put in your mouth and when you already feel full.
- Learn about your food weaknesses so you can take steps in limiting or restricting your intake.
- Don't restrict yourself too much, especially in terms of your favorite foods.
- Try "volumetrics," where you fill up with high-fiber, low-calorie foods right before eating your regular meals.
- Avoid eating meals and snacks directly from the containers so you can control your portions.
- Learn how to deal with stress instead of eating through it.
- Eat a lot of foods which are rich in fiber.
- Don't skip meals.
- Dine frequently with people who share the same health and food goals as you.
- Eat slowly and chew your food thoroughly.
- Try to limit your consumption of alcoholic beverages.
- Give meal planning a try.
- Drink water instead of sugary beverages.

- o Don't focus on "dieting." Instead, focus on following a healthy lifestyle.
- o Set goals and stick with them.

2. Binge Eating

Binge Eating Disorder or BED is one of the most common eating disorders in America and it's a very challenging issue to overcome. People who suffer from this condition tend to eat an unusually large amount of food even if they don't feel hungry. They then feel ashamed and guilty after, making this condition damaging to physical, mental, and emotional health. If you want to overcome your tendency to binge eat, try these strategies:

- o Don't deprive yourself by convincing yourself that you should follow a strict diet.
- o Make sure that you eat meals regularly.
- o Learn "mindful eating," which makes you more aware of what you're eating and how you feel while you're eating.
- o Drink enough water to stay hydrated.
- o Give yoga a try.
- o Remember that fiber-rich foods are your friend.
- o Clean out your home, especially your kitchen.
- o Consider starting your own exercise routine.
- o Never skip breakfast.
- o Make sure that you get enough sleep each night.
- o Try keeping a food journal (more on this later).
- o Talk about your issue with someone whom you know can help you deal with it.

3. Under-eating

On the other side of the spectrum, there are some people who don't eat enough each day. In fact, they eat such small amounts of food that they are starting to damage their health as well. A lot of people who end up under-eating are usually those who try to cut their caloric intake to lose weight. But not eating isn't the answer! If you find yourself struggling with this problem, here are some tips which may help you:

- Instead of skipping meals, learn how to make healthier food choices to help you reach your food goal.
- Don't focus too much on what you need to do to lose weight.
- Focus on following a healthy lifestyle and a clean diet in order to make yourself feel better.
- Keeping a food diary or journal may also be helpful with this issue.
- If you think you need help, consult with a professional.

Chapter 2:
Finding Physical and
Mental Energy

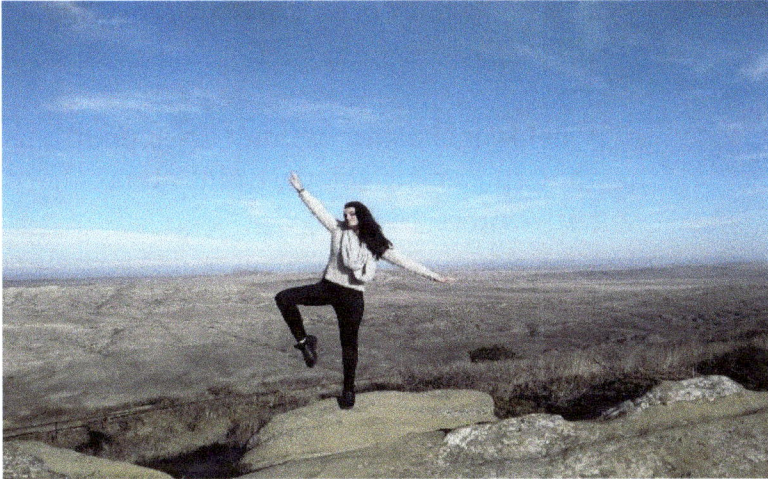

After cleaning up your diet and lifestyle, it's time to find physical and mental energy to keep you going. If you want to be the best version of yourself, someone you love and accept completely, there are a lot of things you must do. To acquire the energy you need, movement and physical activity are key.

Often, health experts claim that exercising for at least half an hour, five time each week can already help you become a healthier individual. But exercising regularly comes with benefits that go beyond having a healthy body, it also helps improve your mental health. Let's look at some of these benefits:

1. **The physical benefits of exercise**

   o It helps your body burn fat at a much faster rate, thus leading to significant weight loss.

- It helps strengthen the body by building muscle tone and mass.
- It helps raise energy levels to improve your agility and performance.
- It helps keep the shape of the body protected as it increases overall muscle strength and flexibility.
- It helps enhance neuromuscular coordination while also developing a stronger skeletal structure.
- It helps make the immune system stronger while improving the gastrointestinal and digestive processes.
- It helps in the management of different disorders such as hypertension, diabetes, cardiovascular disease, and more.
- It helps lower the risk of developing some cancer types.

2. The mental benefits of exercise

- It improves concentration and memory.
- It stimulates endorphin production to help calm the mind as well as reduce the effects of depression and stress.
- It enhances mental agility and self-confidence.
- It plays an important role in controlling discontent thus making it crucial for the process of anger management.
- It promotes high-quality sleep which is crucial for the health and normal functioning of the brain.

How to Remain Physically Active

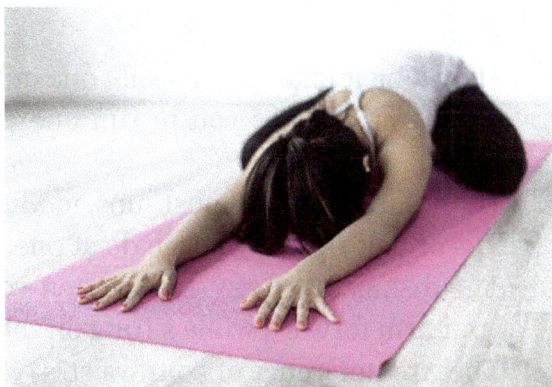

If you want to start living a healthier lifestyle, one of the best things that you can do is to start your own fitness program to ensure that you always remain physically active. This doesn't necessarily mean that you should go to the gym and spend your time there. When it comes to physical activity, go at your own pace. You don't have to be an athlete to become healthy.

In fact, if you can find a physical activity which you really enjoy and which makes you feel good, there's a higher chance that you'll stick with it. Here are some steps for you to follow in order to start your own customized fitness program:

- **Assess your own level of fitness**

  Think about yourself right now and try to assess your fitness level. Do you engage in a lot of physical activities each day or do you spend most of your time sitting down while working? This is the first thing you must do.

  Part of the assessment is to record your baseline fitness scores to have a benchmark to use when you're measuring your progress. In order to get these baseline scores, record the following:

- o Your resting pulse rate.
- o Your pulse rate right after you have walked one mile.
- o How long it takes you to walk one mile.
- o How long it takes you to run one and a half miles.
- o How many standard push-ups, modified push-ups or half sit-ups you can do at one time.
- o The distance you can reach when you stretch your arm forward while sitting on the floor.
- o The circumference of your waist.
- o Your BMI or body mass index.

- **Design your custom fitness program**

  Saying that you'll exercise daily is a lot easier than actually doing it. If you want to solidify your resolve, the best thing you can do is come up with a plan for your fitness program. When you design this program, here are some pointers to keep in mind:

  - o Think about the fitness goals you want to achieve. Setting these goals and making them clear helps you keep track of your progress while staying motivated.
  - o Create a balanced fitness program. Start off slowly and gradually increase the frequency and intensity of your physical activity. This helps your body adjust to this new routine.
  - o Try to find time for physical activity in your daily routine. Although this may be challenging, you can look schedule exercise times as you would schedule your other appointments. If you think it will help, pair your exercise activities with activities you enjoy. For instance, you can take a walk while listening to music,

jog on a treadmill while watching your favorite shows, and so on.

o Vary your physical activities and exercises. This makes it more effective as opposed to doing the same thing repeatedly.

o Make recovery part of your plan. It's never a good idea to push your body too hard as you might get injured or you might start experiencing aches and pains. When you create your fitness program, don't forget to include relaxation and recovery.

- **Assemble all the equipment you need**

  The types of equipment you would assemble depends on the types of physical activities you plan to incorporate into your daily routine. For instance, if you love running or power walking, you must have the right shoes for this. If you don't own a good pair of running or power walking shoes, this is the first thing you must get for yourself.

  If you want to invest in various exercise equipment, make sure to choose those that are fun and easy to use, as well as practical. You can try out the different equipment at fitness centers before you purchase your own personal exercise equipment.

  Finally, you may also want to download a good fitness or activity tracking app on your smartphone to help you with your physical activities. Such apps are very useful because you can keep track of your progress on them. The more you see improvement, the more motivated you will be.

- **Get started!**

  After all the planning, it's time to get started. Remember that this is something you will be doing long-term in order to improve your physical, emotional, and mental health. Although it may seem challenging at first, keep with it, especially if you want to enjoy all the benefits. Here are some things to keep in mind as you start your new fitness program:

    o Start slowly then gradually build up your routine when you think you're ready for more.
    o If you feel like you can't handle the routine at the beginning, break up the activities.
    o When it comes to thinking of exercises and physical activities, be as creative as possible to make it more fun and motivating.
    o Listen to and be aware of your body. If you're feeling dizziness, pain, and other unusual symptoms, rest for a while.
    o Don't take your fitness program too seriously. If you feel like you're pushing yourself too hard, take a break and relax.

- **Keep track of your progress**

  Finally, don't forget to keep track of your progress. You can do this by keeping a fitness journal, a digital diary, or by using a fitness app. It doesn't matter how you monitor your progress; the important thing is that you always keep track of how you're doing.

Motivating Yourself to Keep Going

Now that you have your own custom fitness program, the next thing to do is to make sure that you stick to it. Often, people feel very enthusiastic at the beginning, but they soon lose their motivation to keep going, especially when they don't see or feel immediate results. Nobody said that change is easy. But if you put in the time and effort, the time will come when you will see the fruits of your labor.

No matter how driven you are to become more physically active, you won't start feeling the benefits until you start moving and you learn how to motivate yourself to continue with what you've planned each day. Motivation is a huge part of this process. But how do you keep yourself motivated?

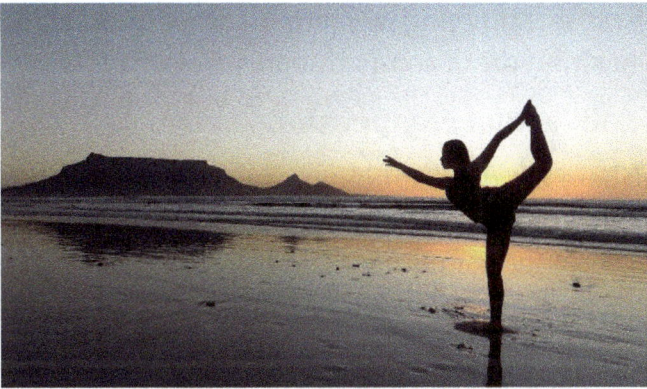

Here are some helpful suggestions for you:

- **Invite someone to take this fitness journey with you**

   Most of the time, we feel more motivated when we're exercising or doing a fun physical activity with a friend. When you're able to find a buddy to workout with, you can encourage and support each other to stick with your plans until you've reached your goals and beyond.

- **Join a fitness club**

   For some people, they feel more motivated when they're part of a group. If you're this type of person, then the best thing for you to do is join a fitness class, a fitness club, or a fitness group. This may help motivate you and it can also help you meet new friends.

- **Start a competition... with yourself**

  This suggestion is especially useful if you are a competitive person. When you compete with yourself, it's like you are pushing yourself to become better each time. Of course, don't forget to listen to your body. You may be so intent on beating your own record that you end up compromising your health. Just as when you're competing with others, you should engage in a healthy sort of competition with yourself.

- **Join actual competitions**

  There are different kinds of fitness competitions you can attend, such as marathons. These are usually held within the community and they're usually a lot of fun! Again, apart from being able to add to your physical activities, you will be able to meet a lot of like-minded people when you join these kinds of competitions.

- **Listen to music**

  Music can be a powerful motivator. When you're feeling down or lazy, try playing some upbeat dance music, preferably those which you really love. Soon, you'll find yourself feeling more energized. You can also turn the TV on while you're doing your physical activity if you think that it will help. You can do push-ups or sit-ups while watching your shows. Pairing your exercise with a fun activity makes it easier to get through it.

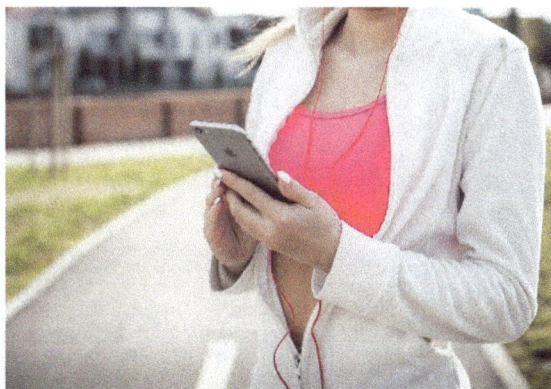

- **Read about people who have succeeded**

Another thing you can do to remain motivated is to read some inspiring success stories. If you're feeling particularly overwhelmed or challenged, go online and search for these stories. There are a lot of them out there. So many people have faced the same challenges at the beginning of their journeys. The important thing is that you want to make a change, so do everything that you can to keep yourself motivated.

- **Never push yourself**

Although this has already been mentioned, it's worth mentioning again. Yes, you want to improve your life by becoming more physically active. But pushing yourself too hard isn't the way to go. If you start feeling discomfort or pain, stop and allow your body to recover. And when you give yourself time off, don't feel guilty about it. Keep in mind that you're trying to learn how to love and accept yourself more. So, do things at your own pace and this will make you feel more inspired in the long-run.

Chapter 3:
Getting Started

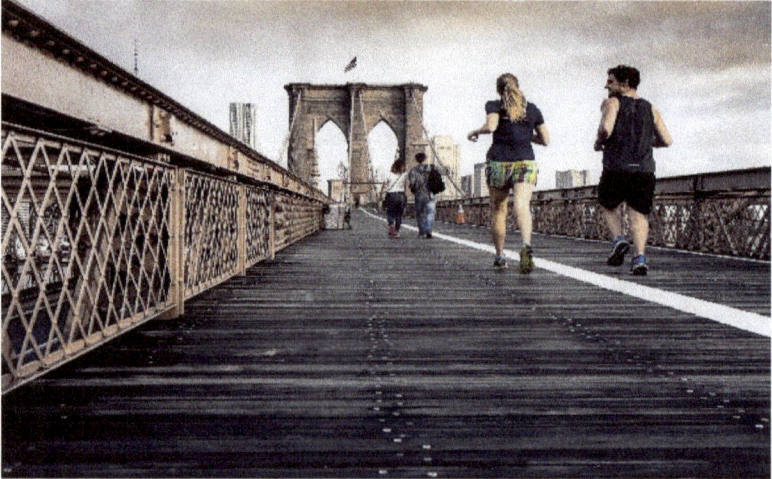

Are you feeling more positive towards yourself yet?

If not, don't worry, we're just getting started. Anyone who plans to improve their life must commit to it. It's not just about saying that you want things to get better, it's more about doing something to initiate that change. For some people, loving themselves isn't an easy task, especially when they lived most of their lives being negative and cynical.

Happiness is a choice and the more you work on having it, the easier this choice becomes. Now, let's help you get started. Although you may not feel happy or satisfied with your body right now, this doesn't mean that you can be. Come up with a plan with achievable and actionable steps to help point you in the right direction. To make it easier for you, let's look at some easy steps to help you with getting started.

Setting Goals

No matter what kind of change you plan to make in your life, the first thing you must do is set goals for yourself. It's very difficult to think of steps to make you love your body more when you don't have concrete goals to look forward to. It's not as simple as waking up tomorrow and telling yourself that "I will love the body I have."

Sure, this might make you feel better for some time, but sooner or later reality kicks in and you're left having to deal with everything else in your life. Then you forget what you told yourself and each time a challenging situation comes up, you go right back to how you previously saw, felt, and thought about yourself.

Setting goals makes it easier for you to plan for what you want and think of steps on how you can get there. The best part is that you don't even have to think of huge or difficult goals! As a matter of fact, it's much more effective to come up with one long-term goal and a few short-term goals to keep you motivated along the way. To illustrate this better, here's an example:

Let's say you feel unhappy or unsatisfied with your body because you feel like you're overweight. This is one of the most common reasons why people don't love their bodies. In this case, you can make a list of goals, such as:

- **Long-term goal: Reach your target weight.**
- **Short-term goals:**
    - Come up with a fitness plan.
    - Learn about the different kinds of healthy diets and lifestyles.
    - Determine which diet or lifestyle suits you.

      ○ Make a plan to follow the diet and lifestyle you've chosen.

These are only a few examples of goals you can set for yourself. As you can see, you would have one long-term goal and a number of short-term goals which will help you move towards your main goal bit by bit. Come up with a list of your own and use that for the next step.

Having a Plan

After you've decided on your goals, it's time to come up with a plan to achieve each of them. This is an effective way for you to have a guide for what you need to do. Anytime you feel overwhelmed, confused, or lost, all you have to do is go back to the plan you've made and see what comes next.

Although some people don't like making plans, this is actually a very helpful way to ensure that you will reach the goals you've set for yourself. Take some time to reflect on these goals and think about how you will be able to reach them. You don't have to treat this step like a chore or something too difficult. Since you'll be the one thinking of the steps, you can make them as simple or as complex as you want them to be.

Using the same example from the first step, let's try to come up with a plan for one of the short-term goals we've mentioned:

- **Goal: Learn about the different kinds of healthy diets and lifestyles**

  There are so many types of diets out there and they all come with their own advantages and disadvantages. Before you can choose which one suits you the most, you need to learn all about them. Here are some steps for you to do this:

- Go online and search for a list of different kinds of diets. Try to find a website that provides a list along with a short description to give you a better idea of what they're all about.
- Make your own list of the diets which seem appealing to you. You should choose 3-5 diets that you think you will be able to follow.
- Now, learn about these diets individually. As you learn more about them, you will have a better idea of what each diet involves and whether it's right for you.
- Narrow down your options to 2-3.

Since your goal here was merely to learn about the different diets, when you reach this step, you're done! The simpler your short-term goals are, the more effortlessly you will be able to achieve them. This is important, especially at the beginning, as it will keep you motivated to move on to the next step until you've finally reached your main goal.

Being Realistic

From the time you decide to embark on a journey towards becoming more loving and happier with your body, you must always remember to be realistic. There's nothing more disheartening than trying to achieve idealistic or impractical goals. Setting such goals would be like setting yourself up to fail, so you may want to rethink your strategy.

Being realistic is easy. All you have to do is think about what you want and what you can do about it. If you don't love your body, reflect on why that is. Are you really unhappy or do you simply feel despondent whenever you try to compare yourself with other people? Are you unhappy because your size doesn't allow you to be as mobile or as agile as you want to be? Are you unhappy because you always feel physically tired and weak? Or are you unhappy because you're not as fit as you want to be?

There are many reasons why people are able to love others with all their heart but aren't able to give themselves that same degree of affection. Whatever your reason is, it's time to start changing this. Because when you think about it, you really won't be able to love others completely unless you learn to love yourself as well.

Going back to being realistic, this mainly applies to the goals you will set for yourself. Go back to the list of goals you created and try to determine if they're realistic enough. Think about your own skills, capabilities, and even the time you have to take the steps to reach those goals. If you think that the goals you've listed down are realistic and doable, that's great! If not, you may have to make a few changes to them in order to make it easier for you to achieve them all.

Knowing How to Adjust as You Go

Speaking of making changes, this is an important part of this last step for getting started. Even though you've spent a lot of time and effort into coming up with your goals and your plans for these goals, that doesn't mean that they're written in stone. This means that if you happen to encounter a challenge along the way, you must also know how to adjust as you go.

There's nothing wrong with challenges and failures. As long as you try your best to overcome them, these hardships will make you stronger and more resilient. In cases where you find it difficult to reach one of your goals, whether it be short-term or long-term, don't be discouraged. Instead, try to think of a way to make an adjustment to your plan or to the goal you have set.

Maybe you had just set a goal which is too difficult for you to achieve at that moment. In that case, what you can do is break down the goal into two or three parts, making it easier to achieve. If the trouble lies in one of the steps in your plan, then adjustment that too. Learn how to be flexible when it comes to achieving your goals. As long as you're working towards these goals, it doesn't really matter how you do it.

Also, learning how to adjust as you go helps you learn to be more accepting of yourself. Instead of feeling bad or berating yourself for not being able to conquer challenges, you simply pick yourself up and find a way to deal with the situation. In doing this, you'll see how easy it is to become more loving and happier with yourself too.

Chapter 4:
The Dos and Don'ts of
Loving Your Body

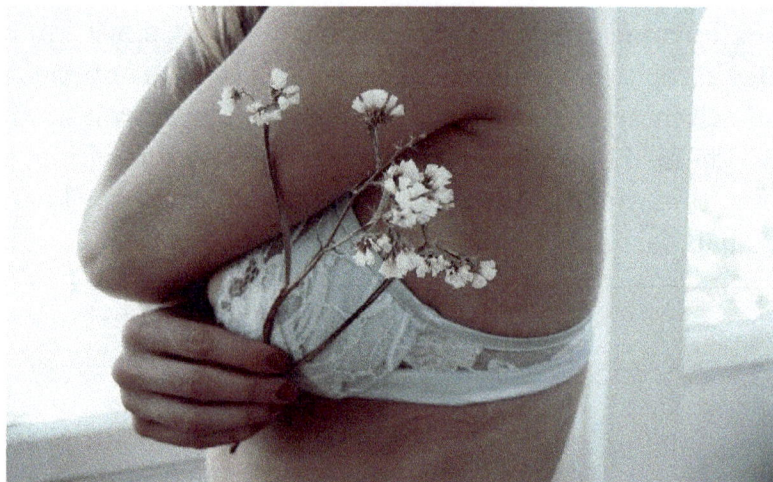

Loving your body is easy. That is, if you know what it really means and what it entails. Think about how you feel about your body right now. Are you happy with it? Is there something which you'd like to change about it? Are you comfortable with your own body?

Some people may say that they love their body but they're not confident about it at all. So, they hide behind layers of clothing while calling this their style. Then when they're on their own and they get the chance to see or feel their body, they feel a sense of discontent or a yearning for something better.

If this situation sounds familiar to you, then maybe you're not happy with your body. Of course, this doesn't mean that fit or slim people are the only ones who are happy with the bodies they have. Sometimes, even the people that others envy want something else. This is the biggest issue when it comes to learning how to love your body. It's not just about achieving the "perfect" body, it's more about accepting the body you have and being comfortable in your own skin.

There are some do's and don'ts that come with loving your body. Although these are general suggestions, you should still try to find what works for you personally. Remember that you are unique, and this means that what may work well for someone else might not work for you in the same way. Therefore, you may have to try a few things and see which ones are suitable for you and which ones you can do without.

Make Sure to DO These Things

We should all take care of our bodies every day. It doesn't matter whether you're completely happy with it or there are things which you would like to change, taking care of your body is an important part of loving yourself. The most basic ways to do this are to learn how to reduce stress in your life, eat healthy foods, exercise regularly, and take a break when you need to.

We all know that taking care of yourself is important. But, doing this isn't easy for everyone. Most people are too busy with the other aspects of their lives to practice self-care. Often, self-care becomes the last thing on our list of priorities. Unfortunately, over time, this can start taking a toll on your body. But loving yourself means that you care for yourself too. Here are some things you should start doing as part of your quest for self-love:

- **DO make adequate sleep a part of your daily self-care regimen**

  Sleep is an essential part of our lives because it has a significant impact on how we feel both physically and emotionally. When you don't get enough sleep, you usually end up being cranky for the whole day. Aside from this, a lack of sleep can also increase your risk of developing a number of health issues.

  You must make sure that you clock in enough hours of sleep each night. If your problem is not being able to fall asleep on time, then you may want to start a bedtime routine. Find ways to wind down before going to bed so your body knows when it's time to go to sleep.

  Part of being able to fall asleep and stay asleep throughout the night is learning how to deal with and reduce stress in your life. If you're able to do this, you won't be troubled by issues which may hinder you from getting a good night's rest.

- **DO prioritize your gut health**

  You may not be aware of it, but the health of your gut influences your overall well-being, health, and vitality. That's why it's important for you to make sure that you always have a healthy gut. A happy and healthy gut makes you a happy and healthy person which allows you to love and appreciate your body more.

- **DO eat right and exercise regularly**

  We've already gone through the importance and benefits of these two things. No matter what kind of good change you want to happen in your life, it will always involve a healthy diet and regular exercise. This is because doing both ensures good health so that you will have the strength and motivation to do everything else.

- **DO prioritize yourself**

  This doesn't mean that you should be selfish in a way that you don't value the other people in your life. It just means that you should start taking better care of yourself just as much as you take care of your partner, your parents or your children. Think about it, if you get sick or if you get to a point where you're so unhappy with yourself that you can't function normally, you're not the only one who will suffer. Make sure self-care is part of your daily routine. And if you need to take a break, do it!

- **DO spend some time outdoors**

  There's really nothing like getting a breath of fresh air. Have you ever seen how happy children are when they are playing outside? This is because they get to do a fun activity in an environment that makes them feel free. Try this out sometime. Take a short stroll around the neighborhood, read a book in your backyard or do something else which relaxes you out in the world. Doing this might even make you feel more connected with your body, your thoughts, and your emotions.

- **DO organize your life**

  Sometimes the problems in our life come from us not being organized enough. We often feel stressed or inadequate because we're not able to deal with things in an organized manner. Try to come up with a plan or a way to bring order into your life. Then you may discover that you actually have free time to do other things which you enjoy, and which make you feel good about yourself.

These are some suggestions for you to start your own self-care routine. There are so many other things you can do which can help you love yourself and your body more. Just as with setting goals and creating plans, find out which works for you and keep doing that.

The DON'TS to Avoid

Of course, if there are things you must do, there are also things which you should avoid. Loving your body doesn't mean that there are no limitations and that you can do no wrong. Self-care doesn't really have to be a time-consuming or challenging process. In fact, the more you do these practices, you may start learning to appreciate and enjoy them. Just make sure you avoid the following:

- **DON'T overdo it**

  Some people indulge in too much self-care and this isn't a good thing. Keep in mind that life is all about moderation and balance. Becoming truly appreciative and fulfilled means that you have to undergo stress and challenges at some point. Don't shy from experiences just because you're not sure about the outcomes and you don't want to feel stressed since you want to "take care of yourself." Never use your self-care practices as a reason to avoid things in life.

- **DON'T forget about the basics**

  What comes to mind when you hear the term "self-care?" These days, for a lot of people, this means going to spas, having massages, using fancy beauty products, and the like. But that isn't all there is. To love your body, never forget about the basics. Staying healthy can be as easy as drinking enough water, eating healthy and balanced meals, getting adequate sleep, and exercising regularly. Simple and basic as these steps are, they will always be highly effective.

- **DON'T spend too much money on your self-care practices**

  Although there's nothing wrong with spending money on yourself, you mustn't use your self-care practices as an excuse to spend too much money. For instance, if you see a cute item of clothing and when you tried it on, you discover that it looks great on you. If you don't normally spend a lot on clothing, this is the perfect time to splurge on yourself. In this example, you want the item and you need it too.

  It is very different to splurge on a bunch of beauty products which claim that they can help improve a part of your body which, incidentally, is the part you feel fairly insecure about. Before spending money on anything, think about it first. This doesn't mean that you should micromanage yourself, it just means that you should be more practical when it comes to your self-care.

- **DON'T just depend on what TV or social media tells you**

  Television and social media are both a blessing and a curse. Through these modern inventions, we can connect with the world in a way that the people in the past only dreamed of. Through television, we're able to learn more about the world and what's happening in it. Through social media, we're able to connect with others and be updated about their lives on a global scale.

  At the same time, both TV and social media can have a negative impact on our lives, especially in terms of how we feel about our bodies and ourselves. All you see on TV and social media are "perfect people" leading perfect lives. Sometimes, they also encourage you to follow a certain lifestyle or a certain diet or even buy certain products so you can be just like them.

Realistically speaking, do you think simply buying something or following a diet will change your life in an instant? Obviously, the answer is no. But when you're feeling unhappy or vulnerable about your body, you tend to believe or *want* to believe everything you see and hear on TV and on social media.

As much as you can, try to avoid this. Don't rely on this information solely. Do your own research, talk to other people, and try to learn as much as you can about the things you want to do or buy before you make a choice. That way, you're prepared for all the consequences of your choice.

- **DON'T believe that "one size fits all"**

Finally, keep in mind that each person is unique. Self-care involves caring for yourself, not for anyone else. Although you may ask advice from other people or read about how you can care for yourself more effectively, it all boils down to you. You have to decide what's best for you, what makes you feel comfortable, and what makes you happy.

Chapter 5:
Shopping and Cooking

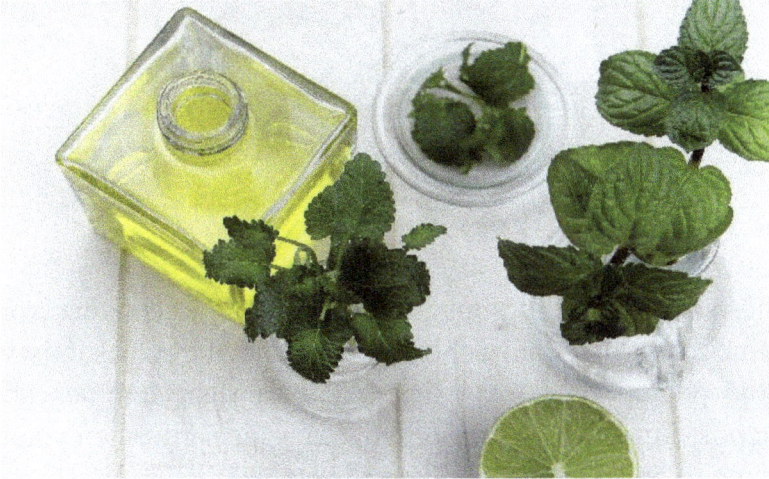

Changing your diet involves more than just ordering different kinds of dishes from restaurants. Since you will be eating most of your meals at home, you must also make changes in your shopping habits and in the way you cook your food.

An important part of loving your body is nourishing it properly. If the diet you're currently following includes a lot of processed, refined, and generally unhealthy options, it's time to start making a new list of foods to shop for. It's also time to start learning how to cook new dishes using those fresh, healthy ingredients you've bought.

The Importance of Cooking from Home Using Healthy Ingredients

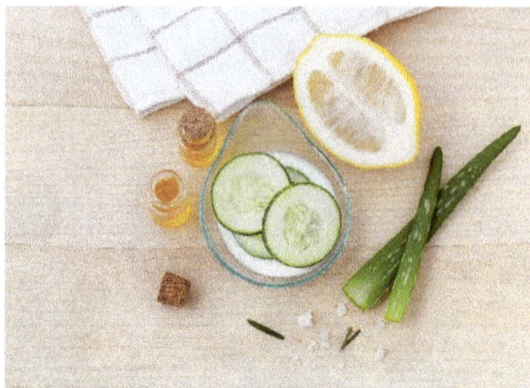

These days, we are so busy with our lives that cooking from home seems like such a chore. This is one of the reasons why most people choose to dine out with their families and friends. But this isn't recommended, especially when you're trying to make changes in your lifestyle. Dining out too frequently or indulging in convenient processed and pre-packaged foods won't help you become a healthier person. These options are also costly and unhealthy.

To keep up with your journey to self-improvement, you should try cooking from home more often. There are many benefits to doing this including:

- **It's healthier**

  Restaurants, fast food chains, and convenience stores may offer ready-made meals, but these are typically high in fats, carbohydrates, sugars, sodium, and calories. Often, they also have very low nutritional content. But if you cook your own food using fresh, whole ingredients you've purchased from your local grocery store, you will be able to get healthier and more nourishing meals.

- **You'll learn more about food**

  The more you cook from home, the more you will be able to learn about food. You'll learn that the food we eat isn't just something to fill your stomach. Food has the potential to inflict pain, cause illnesses, and heal as well. All these effects depend on the kind of food you eat, and you will learn more about this as you explore different kinds of ingredients and recipes.

- **It gives you a new appreciation for food**

  Physically preparing and cooking your own food leads to a new kind of appreciation for what you eat. As you chop, grate, fry, boil, and more, you're able to experience your foods with all your senses. This is very important, especially when it comes to mindful eating. The more aware you are of the food you eat, the more you'll be able to feel how the food affects you and whether this effect is positive or negative.

- **You can control the portions of the food you cook and eat**

  When you order food from restaurants, the dishes usually come in huge portion sizes. So, you can either eat everything on your plate or let the rest go to waste. Neither option is ideal. But when you cook your own food, you will be able to control the portions you put on your plate and whatever's leftover, you can store in your refrigerator for another day.

- **Helps you build healthier habits**

  Learning how to cook your meals from home is an excellent first step to jump-start your healthy diet and lifestyle. There are so many sources where you can find healthy recipes to whip up in your own kitchen. Over time, you will start seeing the value of following a healthier diet which, in turn, may motivate you to start other healthy habits.

- **Safety and cleanliness**

  When you purchase the ingredients yourself, prepare these ingredients, and cook them using your own kitchen utensils, you know that the food you eat is safe and clean. You don't have to worry about getting sick because of poor sanitation or unclean preparation.

- **You'll save a lot of money**

  Finally, cooking from home is also more economical. Rather than spending your money on fancy restaurants and unhealthy processed foods, use it to buy fresh ingredients. The great thing about these is that they are typically cheaper than prepared meals. Then once you get home, you can use these ingredients to whip up healthy and tasty meals.

The Importance of Meal Planning

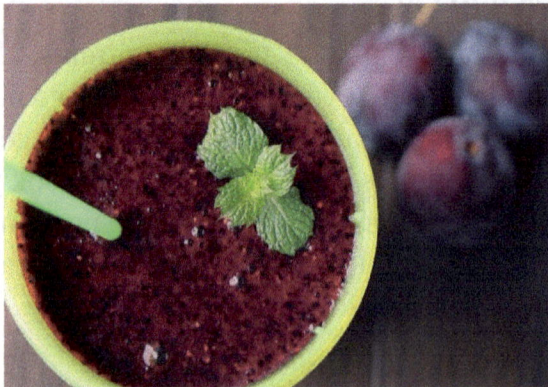

One of the biggest reasons why people don't want to cook their meals from home is that the process is quite time-consuming. When you compare cooking to ordering food from a restaurant, this is definitely true. But have you ever heard about meal planning?

Simply put, meal planning is when you set a specific schedule (usually one day each week) to plan, prepare, and cook your meals for the whole week. For instance, if you don't work on weekends, you may do your shopping on Saturday and your cooking on Sunday, or you may do both on one day. Then, you would store these meals in your freezer or refrigerator. Each day, you would simply heat up the meals you have prepared for breakfast, lunch, and dinner. It's as simple as that!

The great thing about meal planning is that it gives you total control over everything you eat at each meal and for each day. It starts with planning, then budgeting, shopping, preparing, and storing. Although this process may take some getting used to, the more you do it, the easier it gets.

Still not convinced? Here are some reasons that explain the advantages of meal planning:

- **You save time**

   This reason is very appealing, especially for those who always seem to be in a rush. We all have days off, right? Take some time out of those days off for meal planning. The time you spend for this process will allow you to have tasty, healthy, home-cooked meals every day for the rest of the week.

   This means that you won't have to cook your meals individually nor would you have to spend so much money ordering from restaurants. All you have to do is take the meals you have prepared from your refrigerator, heat them up if needed, and enjoy!

   Meal planning also saves you a lot of time at the grocery store. After you've planned your meals for the week, you would write down all the ingredients you need on your shopping list. As you enter the super-market, you know exactly what you will buy, there-fore, you won't spend so much time wandering around while you decide what to buy. And as long as you stick with your list, you won't end up buying un-necessary items that are a waste of money. It's defi-nitely a win-win situation.

- **You eat healthier meals**

  Since meal planning involves cooking your meals from home, both processes share this same benefit. When you plan your meals, you have the freedom to make them as creative, tasty, and healthy as you want. You can mix up your menu to keep things interesting. There are a lot of healthy recipes available online that you can choose from. Create your own compilation of recipes and use these as a reference when planning your meals each week.

- **You save money**

  Again, meal planning helps you save a lot of money which you would have otherwise spent on prepared, packaged, processed, and unhealthy meals. You can save money by purchasing fresh and raw ingredients. You can also save money by limiting the number of times you dine out. This particular reason is why more and more people are becoming interested in meal planning. Who doesn't want to save money, right?

Tips for Meal Planning

As you can see, meal planning is highly beneficial. But if you don't know how to do this, you may feel overwhelmed. Just like any new skill or concept, you need to learn more about meal planning before you start doing it. Also, you should keep practicing meal planning to get better at it. Here are some pointers to start you off:

- **Plan your meals**

  This is an obvious one. The first step in meal planning is the planning itself. Before you go shopping for ingredients, take time to sit down and think about what meals you want to eat for the week. To make it easier and more organized, have two lists with you. One for the meals and the other for the ingredients you need.

  After completing these lists, check your kitchen or pantry compared to the list of ingredients you made. You may discover that you already have some of the ingredients you've written down. In this case, you can cross these items off your list, so you don't purchase them again.

- **Organize your recipes**

  First, you have to search for recipes. A simple Google search will provide you with countless options. If you want to narrow down the options, choose the right keywords. For instance, if you want to look for easy-to-prepare breakfast recipes, use these keywords for your search or if you only want recipes which use plant-based ingredients, then use those keywords. When it comes to searching for recipes online, you have to be as specific as possible if you want to find something in particular.

  After you've printed out all the recipes you find interesting, it's time to organize them. Purchase a binder or a clear book to store all these recipes. That way, you can refer to this file every time you sit down to plan your meals. As time goes by, you can keep looking for and adding new recipes to this book allowing you to mix and match your meals every week.

- **Check for leftovers**

  Before you sit down to plan your meals, check your refrigerator for any leftovers. You may have missed one or two of your meals from the previous week because you dined out or you were too tired to eat your meal before going to bed. No matter what your reason is, skipping meals leaves you with leftovers. In such a case, you can bump up these meals to the start of your week and only plan your meals for the rest of the days.

- **Plan strategically**

  While thinking about your meals, try to think of dishes which share the same ingredients. That way, you don't have to purchase too many ingredients at one time. This also makes it easier to prepare your meals when you only have a few ingredients for different kinds of dishes.

- **Consider making extra**

  The great thing about meal planning is that you can create as many meals as you want when it's time to cook. Another great tip is to make extra and store this in the freezer. That way, if you're not in the mood for the food you planned for a certain day, you have other options. Then you can simply bump up those meals you skipped for another day or for the next week. Just make sure that the meals you bump up to other days don't spoil easily so they won't go to waste.

- **Be flexible**

  Finally, don't take your meal planning too seriously. Allow yourself to have "cheat days" occasionally, especially when you're really craving something. The more you restrict yourself, the more you will feel negatively towards this new change you're trying to implement in your life. Remember to go easy on yourself and give yourself a break once in a while.

Tips for Grocery Shopping

After planning your meals and the ingredients to use for those meals, it's time to hit the grocery store. Even before you start meal planning, it's a good idea to visit the local supermarkets, grocery stores, convenience stores, and farmer's markets to see what they have to offer. That way, you know whether you can make the recipes you've found online or if you can substitute some of the ingredients with the available options. This time, let's look at some valuable grocery shopping tips for you to keep in mind:

- **Always bring your shopping list with you**

  The moment you set foot into the supermarket, you will be faced with seemingly endless choices of food items, from fresh produce to snack items. It's easy to get overwhelmed in supermarkets and it's also easy to start buying impulsively, especially when you don't have a shopping list.

If you recall our first tip for meal planning, it involves creating a list of ingredients you need for the meals you will be cooking. Since you've already made the list, make sure that you bring it with you when you go shopping. That way, you know exactly what to buy so you won't have to go to the other aisles that don't contain what you need.

- **Give yourself some options**

  When you create your list of ingredients, it's also a good idea to give yourself other options in case the ingredients you need aren't available. This saves you a lot of time when you're unable to find the food items you need for your planned dishes. You can check the recipes to see possible substitutes for ingredients and note these down on your shopping list too.

- **Shopping for different food items**

  If you aren't easily tempted and you enjoy going around the entire supermarket, there's nothing wrong with that. Even though you have a list, going around the supermarket gives you an idea or even inspiration for the meals you can plan for the next week. Here are some shopping tips for the different types of food items you may find in the supermarket:

  - When searching for fresh produce, choose different colors. These colors indicate the nutrient content of fruits and vegetables.
  - For pasta, bread, and cereals, go for the ones that are made from whole grains.

- If you plan to continue eating fish, poultry, and meat, make sure to choose fresh fish, skinless poultry, and lean cuts of meat.
- For dairy products, go for unflavored varieties, especially for milk and yogurt products.
- Frozen foods are great, especially for times when you need to prepare a quick meal, as long as you don't rely on them too much.
- Dried and canned foods are alright too as long as you choose products that don't contain high amounts of sugars, sodium, and artificial ingredients.

Chapter 6:
Believe in Yourself to
Reach Your Goals

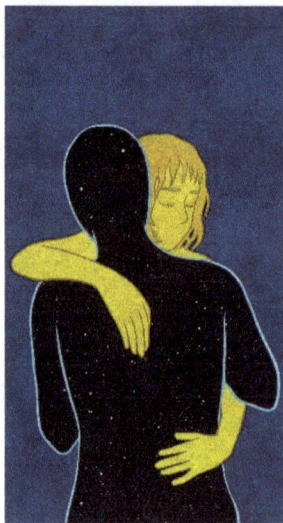

Loving your body goes beyond the physical aspect. This means that you can only truly love the skin you're in when you learn how to believe in yourself as well. Believing in yourself is an important aspect of reaching your goals. However, one thing you need to have in order to do this is the right motivation. Without motivation, you won't be able to keep going.

Too often, people give up on their quest for self-improvement because they lose their motivation. If you don't want to be one of these people, then you must actively look for ways to inspire intrinsic motivation. This type of motivation is far more powerful than the motivation you get from external rewards. Consider these statements when you're feeling unmotivated, stuck, or unwilling to push through with your plans:

- Find something that motivates you no matter what the activity may be.
- Focus on your goals and on the actionable steps which you have made for yourself.
- Change up your routine once in a while so you don't end up getting bored with it.
- Make things fun for yourself so you don't see the steps in your plans as chores or challenges.
- Write down your plans to serve as a physical reminder of what needs to be done.
- Find support from those closest to you in order to stay motivated.
- Reward yourself occasionally, especially after overcoming something particularly challenging.
- Allow yourself to make mistakes and learn from them.

If you keep all these tips in mind, you will find it a lot easier to believe in yourself and stay motivated throughout your journey, and when you start seeing positive changes in your life it will keep you more inspired to keep going. Positivity is important, especially when you're trying to improve your life.

Self-Confidence and Motivation

Motivation is a basic part of our lives. It's powerful enough to influence how and when we perform the tasks we need to do. Motivation is a hypothetical construct utilized in order to describe the external and internal forces that create the direction, intensity, persistence, and initiation of behavior.

Motivation can either be extrinsic or intrinsic depending on where the reward comes from. In general, people who depend on extrinsic motivation aren't as successful in reaching their goals compared to those who depend on intrinsic motivation. Still, extrinsic motivation can have powerful effects on a person, especially at the beginning of their journey.

Self-confidence is one factor that drives motivation. It can either hinder or help a person's performance depending on how much self-confidence the person has and what the task requires. Self-confidence is a person's belief in his own capacity to plan and organize actionable steps needed to produce specific results.

So, how are these related?

A person who has poor self-confidence may find it difficult to motivate themselves to achieve their goals. In fact, they might not even have the confidence to decide to improve their life. People without self-confidence, those who feel broken or defeated might not have the willingness to take that all-important first step.

When you look at it this way, how would such people be able to find the motivation to make their lives better when they don't even think that they can do anything right? If you feel that you lack self-confidence, this should be the first thing you work on even before you start learning to love your body.

Learn more about yourself, what you're good at, and what your strengths are. Doing this will help make you feel better about yourself, thus increasing your self-confidence. Also, you should spend more time with people who love and appreciate you. Think of them as your support system. Having a strong support system goes a long way in terms of building self-confidence. And when you feel like your self-confidence has improved, then you can start looking for ways to improve the other aspects of yourself.

How to Improve Your Self-Confidence

We all need self-confidence in order to succeed. If this is one of your weaknesses, then it's time to start improving yourself. Even if you grew up without self-confidence, there is still hope for you. Self-confidence isn't something you're born with, it's something which you build. Although it would have been better if you grew up with self-confidence, you must work with what you have right now. So, if you're struggling with this, here are some ways to help you build your self-confidence:

- **Practice self-awareness**

  Self-awareness is the basis of self-confidence. Often though, this is overlooked. You cannot take action unless you know yourself and who you really are at your very core. It's important for you to understand all your strengths, weaknesses, dreams, and desires. The more self-aware you are, the more you will be able to build your self-confidence. Here are some self-awareness exercises to try:

  - Take some time for yourself in a room with no distractions. Close your eyes and try to see your life's story through the eyes of those around you. As you do this, try to see how your experiences have molded and influenced who you have become as a person.
  - Start a conversation with your family and your closest friends. Ask them what they think your strengths are as well as what you need to improve on. Ensure them that you're totally open to constructive criticism and that you won't feel bad when they tell you about your weaknesses.

- Try mindful meditation. This is an excellent way to become more aware of your body, your thoughts, and your feelings.

- **Do things that make you happy**

  When you enjoy the things you do, you feel more confident in doing them. Therefore, if you choose to do things that make you happy, the more it will help build your self-confidence. This is why it's a good idea to pair exercising with activities you enjoy such as listening to music and watching TV.

  Even cooking can become a more enjoyable activity while you listen to your favorite tunes. Over time, you won't even notice that you're getting better at the things you're doing because you're having so much fun. Then when you realize that you've improved without realizing it, it will be a huge confidence booster for you.

- **Practice positive visualization and self-talk**

  Negativity has a huge impact on your self-confidence. When you hear other people say mean or derogatory things about you all the time, you might start believing them. When you start internalizing the bad thoughts, words, and actions of those around you, your self-confidence starts to plummet.

  To combat this, you should try practicing positive visualization and self-talk. Positive visualization involves thinking of situations where you succeed. For instance, you can try visualizing yourself already achieving the goals you've set. Try to picture how you look, feel, act, and so on. The more you visualize all these things, the more your subconscious starts working to achieve them.

The same thing goes for positive self-talk. Keep reminding yourself of your strengths and how well you are progressing. The more you encourage yourself, the more confident you will become in your capabilities. Combine these two and you'll start seeing see huge changes in your life.

- **Give journaling a try**

  Starting and maintaining a journal is an excellent way to build your self-confidence. In your journal, you can write down anything that makes you feel good. You can write down your goals, dreams, strengths, and all the other good things in your life. You can also write down the good things you want to have in your life and how you plan to achieve them.

  Maintaining a journal is both cathartic and healthy. Write down any achievements you've made, any breakthroughs, and any challenges. Take some time at the end of each day to add an entry into your journal. This helps build your self-confidence because you're able to see how well you are progressing and how much your life has improved compared to when you started.

- **Don't compare yourself to other people**

  If you want to improve your self-confidence, this is something you should stop *right now*. Keep reminding yourself that you're a unique individual so you should never compare yourself with others. Picture this: you feel insecure about your body and you wish you could change. Now, what do you think will happen when you keep comparing yourself to someone who you think has the "perfect body." Most likely, you'll end up wallowing in self-pity.

This is a dangerous situation because there is a high likelihood that you would just give up and accept defeat. Rather than comparing yourself to others, think about all your capabilities as well as the things you can do to improve your body or whatever it is you want to improve.

- **Be compassionate to yourself**

Finally, learn how to be more compassionate to yourself. The kinder you are to yourself, the more you will have the confidence to tackle tasks head-on. By contrast, the harder you are on yourself, the more likely you'll feel like you cannot really make a difference in your life. So, which situation seems more appealing to you?

Chapter 7:
A Day in the Life of Self-love

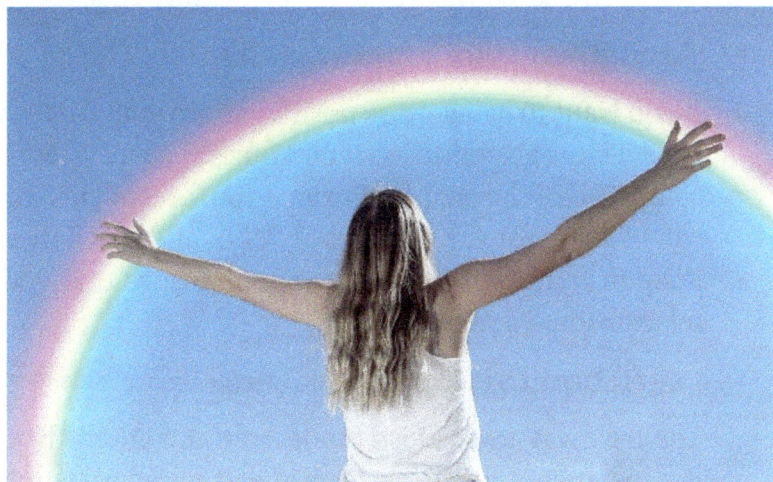

By now you have more than enough information to help you learn how to truly love your body. From everything we've discussed so far, you may notice that it's all about you. That's because learning to love your body also means learning more about yourself.

Caring for your emotional health is just as essential as caring for your physical health. Even though you're able to eat well and exercise regularly, if you ignore your emotional health, you won't be able to truly accept and appreciate all that you are. As a matter of fact, when your emotional health is suffering, you might start experiencing physical symptoms such as chest pains, ulcers, high blood pressure, and more. On the other hand, when you are emotionally stable, you will find it a lot easier to deal with challenges from the small issues to the large events that happen in your life.

Have you ever wondered how you can truly love your body and everything else about yourself? This is a process that doesn't happen overnight. It takes a lot of time, effort, patience, and compassion in order to reach a place where you can genuinely say that you love and accept yourself for who you are. Here are some ways to help you achieve this:

- **Strengthen your support system**

  If you want to bring more positivity into your life, you need a strong support system. Your support system is composed of the people who love you, accept you, and will be there for you in times of doubt and tribulation. Keep in touch with these people to ensure that your relationships don't fade away.

- **Learn how to lessen your fears**

  The best way to do this is to learn more about them. For instance, if you're suffering from a medical condition and you're afraid of how this might affect your life, try to learn as much as you can about it both from your doctor and your own research. The more you learn, the less you'll fear what may happen next because you're prepared for it.

- **Keep moving to lessen your anxiety and improve your mood**

  Remaining physically active is important, especially when you find activities that you actually enjoy. We've gone through the physical and mental benefits of physical activity. But there are social and emotional benefits to this too. When you keep moving, this helps lessen your anxiety and gives your mood a much-needed boost.

- **Have sex!**

  Speaking of enjoyable activities, having sex is an excellent example. When you have sex with someone you love and trust, this level of intimacy helps build your self-worth and your confidence. It makes you feel good physically and it also improves your emotional health.

- **Invest in a new hobby or skill**

  Learning new things or starting new hobbies can improve your life. Investing time in learning a new skill or practicing a new hobby makes you feel fulfilled. The more you practice, the more enjoyable these skills or hobbies will be. Then you'll start seeing a change in your self-confidence as well as how you perceive yourself.

- **Practice yoga or meditation**

  These activities are also highly beneficial in terms of learning self-love. They build your self-awareness, which allows you to focus on your thoughts, feelings, and needs. Aside from this, yoga and meditation are also excellent stress relievers.

- **Avoid overextending yourself**

  It's important for you to learn how to say "no" once in a while, especially when you really can't deal with everything. There's nothing wrong with declining requests or invitations, just make sure to do this in a polite and positive way. Don't assume that people will have ill feelings towards you if you don't say "yes" to them each and every time.

  As long as you explain why you have to decline, chances are they will understand your situation and accept your rejection without feeling bad. Give others a chance so you don't end up overextending yourself.

- **Learn how to manage your time properly**

  Often, you may forget to focus on or prioritize yourself because you always feel like there's not enough time to get everything done. This is especially true when you have a day job and it's particularly stressful. To ease your situation, try to learn how to manage your time better. Come up with a schedule that allows you to take care of yourself while still being able to do all the other important things assigned to you.

A Sample Schedule Which Promotes Self-love

Self-love doesn't have to be just a dream. As you can see, there are several ways for you to nurture love and acceptance for yourself. So, what does a day in the life of self-love look like? Here's a sample schedule/routine which promotes self-love:

- Wake up early so you don't have to rush through your morning.
- Go outside for about 5 minutes or so to breathe in the fresh air, experience the warmth of the morning sun, and just appreciate the moment.
- Take some time to stretch or meditate for about 10 minutes. You may also use this time to practice mind-fulness exercises instead of meditation or stretching.
- Heat up the breakfast you had prepared and stored in the refrigerator for this day.
- Get ready for work. Don't forget to bring your lunch for this day!

- Walk to work if it's not that far. If you need to drive, park your car far from your building so you can still walk from your parking space to your workplace.
- Check all the tasks you need to accomplish for the day. Make a list of all these tasks and arrange them by the level of importance.
- Occasionally, get up and walk around the office. Don't forget to hydrate yourself. You may also strike up conversations with your colleagues once in a while to break the monotony.
- Have lunch. Heat up the packed meal you've brought with you. Converse with your workmates while eating. Share stories, experiences, and laughs.
- Go back to work. Continue with the list of tasks you created when you came in.
- Clock out and go home.
- Have dinner with your family.
- Start your wind-down or bedtime routine.
- Go to sleep at a reasonable hour.

This is a sample schedule you could adopt. As you can see, a lot of the activities involve ways on how you can promote self-love. From eating healthy meals, staying hydrated, interacting with others, having physical activity, and more. There are plenty of ways to deal with your daily life while still taking care of yourself.

You can come up with your own schedule as well and it doesn't have to be the same each day. Make adjustments if you have to and change your routine up to keep things interesting.

A Sample Meal Plan to Go with Your Day

Now that you have a better idea of a schedule you can work with, let's look at a sample meal plan to go with the previous sample schedule. Remember that you would have already prepared all your meals even before the week started. This makes it easier for you to eat regularly since all you have to do is heat up the meals you've planned and prepared. Here's a sample meal plan for you:

- **Breakfast:**

    Pancakes with cream cheese, butter, and syrup (sugar-free)

    Coffee, heavy cream, and sweetener (no carb)

    Breakfast sausage (sugar-free) or bacon

- **Lunch**

    Pancakes with cream cheese this time with ham, cheese, mayonnaise, and spinach or arugula.

- **Snacks**

    2-3 pieces of string cheese or half an avocado sprinkled with salt and pepper

- **Dinner**

    Buffalo wings with blue cheese dressing (sugar-free)

    Celery sticks

- **Dessert (optional)**

    1 serving of chocolate truffles or chocolate mousse

This is just a sample meal plan. The meals you have each day would depend on what kind of diet you have chosen and what you have planned for the week.

Conclusion
It's Time to Start Changing
Your Life!

There you go! A brief but comprehensive guide to help you learn how to love your body and everything else about you. In this book, we have gone through some clever secrets to help you reinvent your life, change your body, and improve your mind. As you may have noticed, all the things we have gone through are focused on you. How you can start your journey, how you can keep yourself motivated, and how you can learn to love and accept who you are as well as the body you have.

Always remember that you can do this! As long as you set goals, make plans, and do whatever it takes to build your self-confidence and self-worth. Start off small and gradually work your way towards your goals. The more you're able to achieve your short-term goals, the more inspired you will be. And if you stick with it, you'll see that your love for your body and yourself has grown significantly since you began this journey of self-improvement. Good luck!

Bibliography

5 steps to start a fitness program. (2018). Retrieved from https://www.mayoclinic.org/healthy-lifestyle/fitness/in-depth/fitness/art-20048269

5 Proven Ways to Build Self Confidence and Take Life Head On - Fearless Motivation. (2018). Retrieved from https://www.fearlessmotivation.com/2017/08/28/9318/

10 Simple Tricks to Make You a Meal Planning Genius. (2016). Retrieved from https://www.lifeasastrawberry.com/meal-planning-genius/

10 TIPS TO MOTIVATE YOURSELF TO LIVE A HEALTHY LIFESTYLE. (2018). Retrieved from http://promiseorpay.com/blog/10-tips-to-motivate-yourself-to-live-a-healthy-lifestyle/

15 Helpful Tips to Stop Binge Eating. (2019). Retrieved from https://www.healthline.com/nutrition/how-to-stop-binge-eating#section15

23 Effective Ways to Stop Overeating. (2019). Retrieved from https://www.healthline.com/nutrition/how-to-stop-overeating

Cheek, E. The Relationship Between Motivation, Self-Confidence and Anxiety - The UK's leading Sports Psychology Website. (2019). Retrieved from https://believeperform.com/performance/the-relationship-between-motivation-self-confidence-and-anxiety/

Crichton-Stuart, C. The top 10 benefits of eating healthy. (2018). Retrieved from https://www.medicalnewstoday.com/articles/322268.php

Dave, C. Mental And Physical Benefits Of Exercise. (2016). Retrieved from https://www.huffpost.com/entry/mental-and-physical-benefits-of-exercise_n_57d6341be4b0f831f70722f8

Davis, T. Self-Care: 12 Ways to Take Better Care of Yourself. (2018). Retrieved from https://www.psychologytoday.com/us/blog/click-here-happiness/201812/self-care-12-ways-take-better-care-yourself

McCarthy, M. How Journaling Can Boost Your Self-Confidence. (2019). Retrieved from https://www.mindbodygreen.com/0-5139/How-Journaling-Can-Boost-Your-SelfConfidence.html

Morin, A. 5 Ways to Start Boosting Your Self-Confidence Today. (2019). Retrieved from https://www.verywellmind.com/how-to-boost-your-self-confidence-4163098

Orenstein, B. 10 Ways to Boost Your Emotional Health Through Improving Your Self-Esteem. (2017). Retrieved from https://www.everydayhealth.com/emotional-health/10-ways-to-boost-emotional-health.aspx

Physical Activity: Keeping Motivated | Nutrition Australia. (2019). Retrieved from http://www.nutritionaustralia.org/national/resource/physical-activity-keeping-motivated

Rosenberg, M. The Do's and Don'ts of Self-Care | Bella Grace Magazine. (2019). Retrieved from https://bellagracemagazine.com/blog/the-dos-and-donts-of-self-care/

Self-esteem and Motivation - Maslow's Hierarchy of Needs. (2017). Retrieved from https://www.psychology-noteshq.com/maslowhierarchyofneeds/

The 4 Fallacies of Undereating - and How to Overcome This Negative Thinking - Leanness Lifestyle University. (2019). Retrieved from https://lluniversity.com/the-4-fallacies-of-undereating-and-how-to-overcome-this-negative-thinking/

The Dos and Don'ts of Self-Care - College Fashion. (2018). Retrieved from https://www.collegefashion.net/college-life/self-care-dos-and-donts/

The Importance of Meal Planning: 3 Reasons to Meal Plan Weekly. (2019). Retrieved from https://projectmealplan.com/importance-of-meal-planning/

The Top 10 Home Cooking Health Benefits. (2016). Retrieved from https://www.healthfitnessrevolution.com/top-10-health-benefits-cooking-home/

Valente, L. 7 Tips for Clean Eating. (2019). Retrieved from http://www.eatingwell.com/article/78846/7-tips-for-clean-eating/

Wagner, G. 25 Ways to Make Time for Fitness. (2011). Retrieved from https://experiencelife.com/article/25-ways-to-make-time-for-fitness/

Zelman, K. 10 Tips for Healthy Grocery Shopping. (2019). Retrieved from https://www.webmd.com/food-recipes/features/10-tips-for-healthy-grocery-shopping#1

Zeratsky, K. Clean eating is more than washing your hands. (2019). Retrieved from https://www.mayoclinic.org/healthy-lifestyle/nutrition-and-healthy-eating/expert-answers/clean-eating/faq-20336262

INTERMITTENT DIET FOR WOMEN OVER 50

The Complete Guide for Intermittent Fasting Diet & Quick Weight Loss After 50, Easy Book for Senior Beginners, Including Week Diet Plan + Meal Ideas

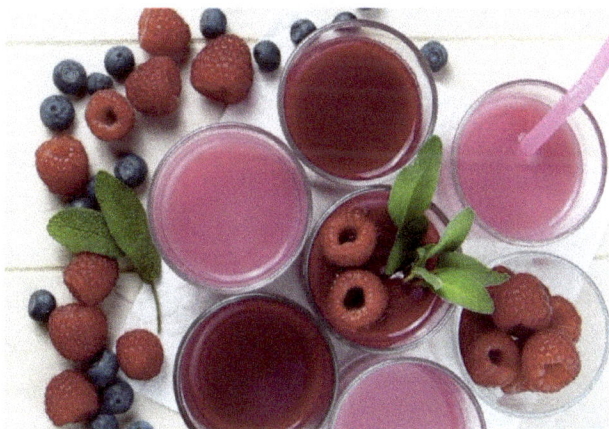

Dr. Gillian Keys Pomroy, Dr. Anna Bernardi

Introduction

When a woman approaches a certain age, her body starts changing as the aging process kicks in. Women over fifty become high-risk targets for various health issues and start to find it harder to maintain their weight.

There has been scientific interest in intermittent fasting as research has started to uncover the numerous benefits of it. Post-menopause causes many changes in a woman including increased belly fat, depression, muscle pain, and joint pain. Women are moreover at more considerable risk for diabetes and cardiovascular disease. These are just a few of the symptoms that can be associated with a metabolic syndrome which is closely related to insulin resistance and prediabetes.

Research has shown that intermittent fasting in women over fifty could possibly reduce the risk of diabetes and may ease muscle and joint pain, especially lower back pain. It could, in addition, produce a positive anti-aging effect which is an added bonus along with better weight control to cut down on belly fat.

Chapter 1:
Introduction to the Intermittent Fasting Diet

Before you start any diet or drastically change your eating pattern, it is always advisable to seek the advice of a medical professional. This is especially true if you have an existing condition, as when there is fasting involved it may interfere with your medication or health.

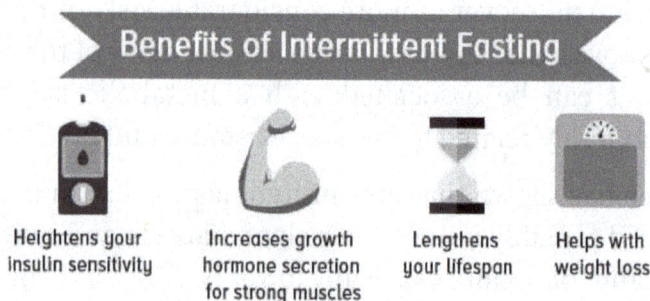

Benefits of Intermittent Fasting

Heightens your insulin sensitivity

Increases growth hormone secretion for strong muscles

Lengthens your lifespan

Helps with weight loss

What is the Intermittent Fasting Diet?

Intermittent fasting (IF) is when a person refrains from eating during certain hours of the day. During the hours that the person is not fasting, they eat a healthy, regimented diet. The intermittent fasting diet is not so much of a diet but a lifestyle change.

Some of the more popular intermittent fasting methods are two to three days a week, alternate days, or daily during set hours. The thing about the intermittent fasting diet is that there is no need for counting calories, macronutrients, or cutting down on certain foods.

There are no set rules other than not eating certain set rules, and you can eat what you like during the time window in which you are not fasting. During the time when you are fasting, you can drink water, tea, and coffee.

Intermittent fasting is a diet that can be used to lose weight, enhance body composition, and decrease body fat. It has been known to have a lot of other health benefits, especially for women in middle age.

Intermittent fasting (IF) is an eating pattern that cycles between periods of **fasting** and eating. It doesn't specify which foods you should eat but rather when you should eat them. In this respect, it's not a diet in the conventional sense but more accurately described as an eating pattern

History of Intermittent Fasting Diet

The father of modern medicine, Hippocrates of Cos, who lived between 460 BCE to 375 BCE, practiced fasting. Fasting an ancient method of healing along with apple cider vinegar. Plutarch was an ancient Greek historian and a writer, he also wrote about fasting rather than using medicine. Even Aristotle and his mentor Plato practiced and believed in fasting. (Fasting — A History Part 1, n.d.)

Fasting has been called the 'physician' within as all animals as well as humans tend to turn away from food when they are sick. If you have ever been really sick you will know that the last thing you think of is food. It is as if fasting is ingrained into a person's DNA, a natural instinctive reaction to sickness as old as time.

After a large meal, the body reduces blood flow to the brain as it pushes more blood to the digestive system to help it digest a large meal. Fasting was thought to improve cognitive abilities by the ancient Greeks. But it was not only the ancient

Greeks and great philosophers that believed in fasting but the founder of toxicology, Philip Paracelsus did too.

Fasting has been used for many other reasons besides medical or losing weight as well. It has also been used for spiritual purposes, religious purposes, purification, cleansing, and to make statements for a cause.

Fasting has been around for many years and will be around for many more years as scientists have now started to take an interest in its many benefits. Our ancient ancestors that were hunter-gatherers had to go out looking for food each day. Sometimes there was no food to be found and so they would go for long periods without eating. As a result, the human body evolved and adapted to be able to go without food for days at a time.

The body functions better when it has been deprived of food for a couple of hours as it gives it a chance to do some in-house cleaning.

Chapter 2:
Types of Intermittent Fasting

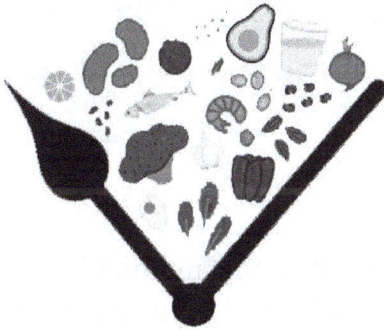

There are different types or methods of intermittent fasting that can be quite effective. The trick is finding out which is the best one for you that suits your needs and lifestyle.

The More Popular Types of Intermittent Fasting Methods

Fasting has periods where you do not eat and then periods called cycles, patterns, or eating windows where a person can eat. The following methods are the most effective for weight loss and are the easiest fasting cycles to follow.

16:8 Intermittent Fasting Method

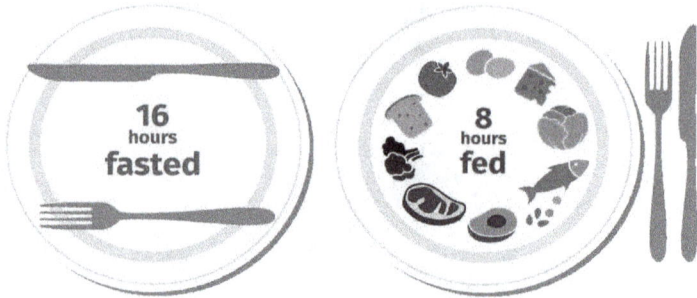

The 16:8 intermittent fasting method is also known as the 8-hour diet as you fast for 16-hours a day and have an 8-hour a day eating window. This method is used by a lot of celebrities and top business people as well as being a popular trending diet on social media.

It is used to help lower the risk of contracting a chronic disease, aids in weight loss, and helps with mental acuity. There is a risk with this type of diet as well as it can lead to overeating within the limited time window if a person does not eat correctly. This is because there is no actual diet or restrictions on what you eat or how much you eat during that time window.

During the 16-hours of fasting a person can consume nothing but unsweetened beverages such as water, tea, or coffee. You should not be consuming fizzy drinks, alcohol, or any other sweetened beverages because they are not healthy for you. They can also lead to health problems because of what goes into those kinds of beverages.

During the 8-hour eating windows, a person is free to eat what they please. Most people who do the 16:8 fasting method find it easier to fast during the evening and through breakfast the next day. Leaving their 8-hour eating window to start at around noon or one o'clock. In order to get the full benefits of an intermittent fasting diet, it can be beneficial to follow a diet plan that suits you. A lot of people will follow diets such as the keto meal plan, weight watchers, low-carb diets, and so on.

The diet you choose should be one that is beneficial to you and caters to your eating needs. What you do not want to do when you are trying to reap the benefits of intermittent fasting is to fill yourself up on empty carbs and sweets. Rather make the most out of your eating window and eat healthily.

This intermittent fasting method is not really for beginners and if you would like to try it you should try a modified version of it. Maybe go to 12:12, fast for 12 hours and eat for 12 hours on a healthy eating plan. Only fast with this method no more than twice a week when you first start with intermittent fasting.

5:2 Intermittent Fasting Method

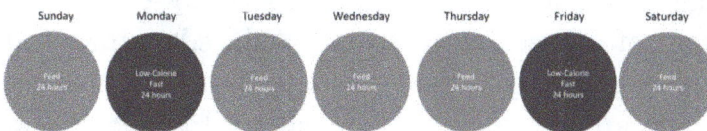

The 5:2 diet is currently the most popular and practiced method of intermittent fasting and is known as the fast diet. Michael Mosley, a British journalist who was diagnosed with type 2 diabetes in 2012 was the one who popularized this method. He managed to turn his life around by losing 26.5 pounds in 12 weeks which helped him get his type 2 diabetes under control.

Throughout our lives, we are told that breakfast is the most important meal of the day. But who says it has to be eaten as soon as we get up or grab something as we rush out the door to start the day? Michael Mosley developed the 5:2 diet believing that a person needs to give their body a rest from food.

The belief of the diet is that when a person goes without food for more than 10-hours the body goes into what is called negative protein or nitrogen balance. When this happens, the body starts to consume and get rid of old proteins and does not produce new ones. When the body does not receive enough or quality protein it starts to consume what it can find and switches the body to cell repair mode.

An early supper and late breakfast are a good way to give the body a chance to completely clean itself out and repair what needs to be repaired. On the 5:2 diet, a person will eat a normal healthy diet for five days of the week. The other two days they will be on a calorie-restricted diet of 500 to 600 calories a day.

A person can choose the two days of the week that best suits them as long as there is at least one to two days in between fasting days. For instance, fast on a Tuesday, eat the normal number of calories required on Wednesday, then fast on Thursday or Friday again. On fasting days, a woman should consume around 500 calories and try to have two small meals for the day. The best eating plan is to have a late breakfast and an early supper to get the best results.

On eating days, a proper, healthy diet should be followed in order to lose weight and enjoy other health benefits of the diet along with regular exercise.

Alternate Day Fasting (ADF) Method

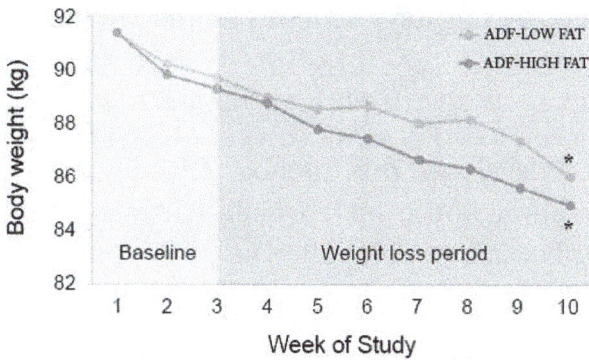

Alternate day fasting or ADF is a fasting method done over a 48-hour period. A person will fast for 36-hours (a day and a half) then eat normally for the 12-hour eating window. Of course, non-sweetened beverages such as water, tea, and coffee with no sugar can be drunk but nothing else during the 36-hours.

During the 12-hour eating window, people can eat a healthy normal diet or anything they want. There is a more popular version of this fasting method where people eat within a certain time period and may consume up to 500 calories. Dr. Krista Varady brought out the "Every Other Day Diet" after studying the alternate-day fasting method.

Beginners to fasting methods find this intermittent fasting diet to be the easiest to maintain. There have been some studies that show this method to be most effective for middle-aged women in losing and controlling their weight. Other studies have shown that it may be able to reduce inflammation markers as well as belly fat in for those who are obese.

The alternate-day fasting method has shown to work with or without a low-fat diet but is most effective when combined with regular exercise. In order to stop or reduce compensatory hunger, the modified version of this fasting method is the most recommended. Eating 500 calories a day at a certain time on fasting days with this method reduces hunger.

Eat Stop Eat Intermittent Fasting Method

Brad Pilon developed this method of fasting after doing research on how it affects metabolism. The eat stop eat method of fasting became popular after he wrote his popular book, *Eat Stop Eat.*

This fasting method requires a person to have two days a week when they fast. These days must not be consecutive days though and should have at least one to two eating days in between.

It sounds a bit painful as a person has to commit to fast for a full 24-hours. For instance, a person could choose Monday and Thursday as their fasting days. This ensures that there are two full days in between their fasting days. Choose time to start fasting from Monday which could be at 10 am which gives you time to eat a good breakfast before beginning your fast.

The fast would then end at 10 am on Tuesday where a person can indulge in a good breakfast. They would eat their normal diet from 10 am Tuesday until 10 am Thursday when they would start to fast again. The fast would stop at 10 am Friday and for the rest of the weekend, the person gets to eat their normal diet.

Although there are no actual dietary requirements for non-fasting days, it is highly recommended to follow a healthy diet. Or at least make healthy food choices and choose foods that have slow-releasing carbs to eat just before starting the fast.

No matter what fasting method a person chooses, it is imperative that they keep themselves well hydrated. Water is always the best solution although an unsweetened coffee or tea can be a nice change.

The Warrior Diet

The warrior diet is quite a strict intermittent fasting method as it follows a 20-hour restricted calorie intake diet and a 4-hour unrestricted diet window per day. This diet is based on the habits of human ancestors that would go hunting and gathering during the day. This would be for most of the day starting in the early hours of the morning to return when the sun was going down. It was during these few hours before they slept that they would eat.

The warrior diet is based on fasting during the night and into the next day until dinner time. Then for 4-hours it is recommended that a person eats nutrient-dense foods although there is no actual limit to what a person can eat during this window. It is, however, advisable to eat good foods such as lots of whole-foods. Unprocessed foods are the foods to aim for on this diet and the good news is you don't have to count calories for 4-hours.

One Meal a Day (OMAD) Diet

This is not the fasting method recommended for beginners and it should not be taken lightly. Before going on this diet, a person should first check with their medical advisor as it is a 23:1 fasting method. This means that a person cannot consume any calories for 23 hours of the day and only has a 1-hour eating window in which to eat.

Before trying this fasting method, a person should learn the best times of day to eat. They should also learn what the best foods are to eat within the 1-hour eating window. They should also only do it once or at most twice a week unless they really know what they are doing.

It does, however, offer rapid weight loss and is not too hard to follow. There is also no need for calories to be counted on the diet. In the 1-hour eating window, a person can eat any food they want. Once again healthy food choices are always the best option.

Chapter 3:
The Benefits of Fasting for Women Over 50

Studies have shown that intermittent fasting may be extremely useful for postmenopausal women to aid in maintaining their weight. There are quite a few benefits to intermittent fasting for middle-aged women or women that are going through menopause no matter their age.

#1:
Fat Loss

#2:
Improved
Cognitive Function

#3:
Lower
Inflammation

#4:
Lower Blood
Pressure

#5:
Blood Sugar
Control

#6:
Better Metabolic
Health

#7:
Longevity

Why for Women Over 50?

Women who approach post-menopause (and sometimes even as early as pre-menopause) tend to start accumulating belly fat. They will start noticing their metabolism get slower. They may also start feeling aches and pains in their joints. Their sleep patterns start to get completely out of routine leaving them feeling exhausted all the time. Then there is the weight gain and also a higher risk of developing chronic diseases like cancer, diabetes, and heart disease that could lead to heart attacks.

There is also the risk of neurodegenerative diseases, stroke, and a constant feeling of fatigue. Intermittent fasting has been known to reset a person's internal balance. This, in turn, boosts their external appearance, energy levels, and cuts down on stress as they control their weight.

Why Should Women Choose the Intermittent Fasting Diet?

Intermittent fasting has become a very popular healthy lifestyle trend, and for good reason. It offers many health benefits as well as improves a person's state of mind and encourages an all-round feeling of well-being.

Benefits of Intermittent Fasting for Women Over 50

INCREASES

- The intensity of the fat burning stage for Keto adapters
- Leptin levels to reduce overeating
- Insulin and leptin sensitivity (lowers risk of cancer, heart disease, and diabetes)

DECREASES

- Weight gain and metabolic damage
- Inflammation and oxidative stress
- Reduces insulin resistance
- Cholesterol levels
- Speed of aging process

When women get to 50 and over, their skin will start to show signs of age. They may find their joints start to ache for no reason, and suddenly belly fat accumulates as if you have just given birth. There are so many creams, diets and exercises on the market to tighten the skin and try to help. The fact is, they may work to a certain point but then the body hits a shelf, and nothing seems to push a person past it. This boils up frustration making women look into the more drastic and very expensive alternatives like surgery. Which in itself poses so many more dangers and risks for women of 50 and over.

A person does not need to go under the knife or starve themselves to reboot their system or change their shape. Intermittent fasting is a much cheaper and less risky way to do this and there is no need to make any drastic eating habit changes either. Well, you may need to make a few adjustments like cutting out junk food and eating healthier. But once again the diet a person follows is their personal choice and depends on how serious they are about becoming healthier.

Some health benefits of intermittent fasting for women over 50 include:

Activating Cellular Repair

Fasting has been known to kick start the body's natural cellular repair function, get rid of mature cells, improve longevity, and improve hormone function. All things that tend to take a battering as people age. This can alleviate joint and muscle aches as well as lower back pain. As the cells are being repaired and damage undone, it helps with the skin's elasticity and health too.

Increase Cognitive Function and Protects the Brain from Damage

Intermittent fasting may increase the levels of a brain hormone known as a brain-derived neurotrophic factor (BDNF). It may equally guard the brain against damage like a stroke or Alzheimer's disease as it promotes new nerve cell growth. It also increases cognitive function and could effectively defend a person against other neurodegenerative diseases as well.

Weight Loss

When people have belly fat, it can cause many health problems that are associated with various diseases as it indicates a person has visceral fat. Visceral fat is fat that goes deep into the abdominal surrounding the organs. Belly fat is terribly hard to lose, especially for an aging woman. Intermittent fasting has been known to help reduce not only weight but inches of over five percent of body fat in around twenty-two to twenty-five weeks (Barna, 2019).

Alleviates Oxidative Stress and Inflammation

Oxidative stress is when the body has an imbalance of antioxidants as well as free radicals. This imbalance can cause both tissue and cell damage in overweight as well as aging people. It can also lead to various chronic illnesses like cancer, heart disease, diabetes, and also has an impact on the signs of aging. Oxidative stress can trigger the inflammation that causes these diseases.

Intermittent fasting can provide your system with a reboot, helping to alleviate oxidative stress and inflammation in a middle-aged woman. It also significantly reduces the risk of oxidative stress and inflammation for those overweight or obese.

Slow Down the Aging Process

As intermittent fasting gives both the metabolism and cellular repair a reboot it offers the potential to slow down aging.

It may even prolong a person's lifespan by quite a few years especially if following a nutritious diet and exercise regime alongside intermittent fasting.

Chapter 4:
Balancing Hormones and Boosting Energy

The endocrine system is the body's system that produces hormones. Hormones are potent chemicals that convey messages through the body to regulate certain processes. Hormones are needed for growth, fertility, metabolism, the immune system, and a person's mood or behavior.

Hormones

As we age our hormones change and our body produces more of some, less of others. Hormones are produced in accordance with the person's stage of life. For example, a teenager's hormones are produced to get them through puberty. The following stage of development for the human body where hair starts to develop in strategic places. A woman's body changes and starts to get ready for the subsequent stage, which is to produce offspring.

During pregnancy, the body produces the human chorionic gonadotropin (HCG) hormone. As well as human placental lactogen (HPL) hormone, estrogen, and progesterone. As most people know, women seem all over the place both physically and emotionally when they are expecting. Now you know why with all these extremely potent chemicals being produced.

Women go through perimenopause usually during their mid-forties. At this stage, the body's estrogen production starts to slow down until they go through menopause. During menopause, the body stops releasing eggs which means a woman is no longer able to reproduce.

Most women will go through menopause between the ages of fifty-one to fifty-two. It can last anywhere from one to three years and the symptoms of menopause can include:

- The menstrual cycle has stopped for a year or more.
- Problems sleeping.
- Bad night sweats that can drench a person.
- Uncomfortably dry or itchy skin that actually feels like you have a thousand ants crawling on you.
- Problems with urination like releasing little drops when sneezing, problems urinating, and incontinence issues.
- Urinary tract infections or dryness which leaves a burning sensation.
- Decreased libido and disinterest in intimacy.
- Some women experience varying degrees of lethargy.
- Hot flashes that cause a person to feel like the doors of hell have opened in front of them. These come on suddenly with no warning at any time or place during the day.

Some women will experience all of these symptoms, some of them, and others may get them more mildly or not at all. Menopause and its symptoms are a lot like being pregnant without giving birth at the end. The hormones or lack thereof, affect each woman differently. It wholly depends on how your body adjusts to the current phase in its lifecycle.

It is vital to try and balance your hormones. One hormone which increases when practicing intermittent fasting is the growth hormone. As soon as a person stops eating for long enough, the body starts to produce this hormone. It is the hormone sent out to repair tissue and is typically called the fountain of youth hormone due to its reparative qualities. While it doesn't do much to change menopause, it will help slow down the aging process and help you retain muscle. It also helps with weight loss, and intermittent fasting has been shown to almost double this hormone in the body.

During menopause, two hormones that become imbalanced are melatonin and cortisol. These are the hormones that need to be in sync, as melatonin helps a person sleep and enjoy good quality sleep. While cortisol is the hormone that helps a person wake up, feel alert, and keep the mind clear. An imbalance of these two hormones is usually due to a health problem, anxiety, stress, and menopause. Intermittent fasting along with proper nutrition may aid in the production and balance of these two hormones.

Homeostasis is the term used for hormone balance and it is vital for optimum health. To be successful with an intermittent fasting program, you also need a nutritious diet. Once a woman reaches fifty it is imperative to live a healthy lifestyle to ensure you enjoy your golden years in peak form.

Women over fifty should strive to:

- Eat well but healthily and make smarter food choices.
- Fast within their comfort zone and make it a part of their life.
- Take supplements to ensure they are getting enough vitamins and minerals.
- Take care of their skin by implementing the proper treatments in or out of the sun.
- Wear protection in the heat when outside. Wear a hat to cover your face and neck. Wear sun protection, although a good 15 minutes of direct sunlight will increase vitamin D.
- Exercise at least two to three times a week, more if you are able to.

- Most importantly drink lots of water.

Energy

Hormones can equally affect a person's energy levels. During menstrual cycles, energy levels have been known to spike and rise due to increased levels of estrogen. But after the menstrual cycle, the levels of estrogen drop quite drastically causing lethargy. As women reach menopause and estrogen levels start to drop, women feel less energetic and extremely tired.

Another hormonal culprit that contributes to a menopausal woman's lack of energy is progesterone. This hormone declines with age and is one of the reasons middle-aged women have problems sleeping. Progesterone is used to induce ovulation in younger women, but it also promotes sleep. Obviously, a woman going through middle age no longer has need of ovulation, so her body does not produce as much as it used to.

Although they do not produce it in the amounts a man does, a woman's body also produces testosterone. Testosterone performs a significant part in the production of red blood cells in the body. Red blood cells are the cells that transport oxygen around the body which is a much-needed component in the promotion of energy. As with many other hormones, menopause limits the production of testosterone as well.

High-stress levels will cause an increase in cortisol, which as discussed in the previous section, you will know keeps a person awake. This affects sleep patterns, which is just another added factor causing a lack of energy due to feeling tired. It will also have an impact on a woman's mood and leave them feeling horrible.

There are ways to increase energy levels but the first step to take is to measure your hormone levels. This can be done by your medical advisor, a registered clinic, or there are home tests you can buy at the drugstore. Ask a pharmacist what the best and most reliable brands are. Once you know what you are dealing with there are a few methods you can try to increase energy levels.

Never try hormone replacements or balancing hormones without the advice of a medical professional. If you are not on any medication or have any pre-existing medical conditions you can try one of the following tips:

- Ask your doctor, nutritionist, or pharmacist to recommend a good quality multi-vitamin. Make sure you fall into a routine of taking them.
- Slowly change your diet to one that offers more nutrition and agrees with your system. As you age you will find foods that you may no longer be able to eat.
- Find a quiet time to take ten to fifteen minutes to meditate, clear your mind, and learn the art of breathing. Tibetan monks have practiced *anapanasati,* which is mindfulness through breathing.
- Get enough good quality sleep. You may need to make some adjustments to your bedroom. Make sure your pillow is supporting your head and that your mattress is doing the same for your body. Take all electronics out of your room, if you use your mobile phone for an alarm make sure it goes into sleep mode. Instead of a TV, make room for a chair to curl up in and read. Reading before bed is a great way to unwind and slip into another world to clear your mind. Try not taking naps during the day.
- Get in some exercise at least once a day, twice if you can manage it. It does not mean you have to go running a marathon or do the Tour de France. Go for a walk, do some gardening, or take a gentle bike ride and look at the scenery.

- Find a new hobby or take up an old one you had put aside. If you engage your mind, you will automatically gear your body up for action.
- There are supplements and certain foods to naturally boost your energy. Whatever you do, do not try highly caffeinated drinks, or other such types of energy boosters you find in a supermarket.

By now you will know the next bit of advice is going to be — drink lots of water. It is a great cure for a whole lot of things including lethargy. If you want to get a little extra boost, try using an icepack on your Vagus nerve in your neck for a minute at a time.

Chapter 5:
Definitive Weight Loss and Increased Mental Clarity

Clean eating, movement, breathing, and fasting have been known to stimulate weight loss as well as clear the mind.

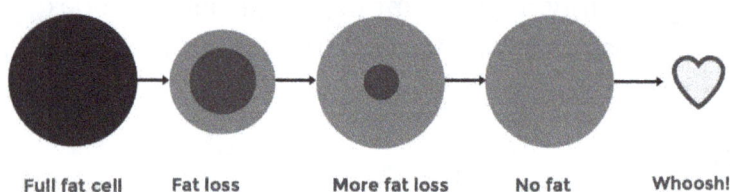

Full fat cell   Fat loss   More fat loss   No fat   Whoosh!

Weight Loss

Losing weight is a mindset really. You have to be motivated to want it and be prepared to do it. Like anything else in life, you have to be mentally prepared for it and want it badly enough to follow through. There are many roadblocks in life and one of the biggest we have to overcome are our own mental roadblocks.

One of the biggest things that hold us back is fear, even if we do not realize we actually fear something. Actual fear is easier to overcome as more often than not we know it is some ingrown irrational state of mind that makes us fear. Like a fear of heights may be a fear of falling from that height and not the actual height itself.

Instead of working our way through it, we simply avoid it, or cower somewhere in the middle of a crowd and peek out at the amazing world from above. It is easy to hide from our fears these days. As the internet allows us to travel, get to the top of the highest mountain, or be who we want to be. We can do all this safely through our screens where we know we have nothing to fear.

Losing weight, getting fit, and being healthy is no different. Before the internet, a person would have to go out and research things like fasting. You actually had to face a person, look them in the eye and have them assess you.

Most fasting for weight loss programs would need to be done through a trained professional. These days all the information you want is on the internet at your fingertips. You can gather it, do all the leg work, and sort out your way forward. The trick is, to have the fortitude to actually start the program and stick with it to reach your goals.

Unlike a monitored weight-loss and fast program, the only person monitoring your program is you. So you have to be both the antagonist and protagonist of your new lifestyle change. You are the one that will need to motivate, monitor, and maintain your program. There is not going to be any gold stars or pats on the back when you do reach your targets.

What you will have instead is a feeling of accomplishment along with starting to feel and look great. You have to be happy with that and realize the only one you need to impress is you. The only one benefiting from your new lifestyle change is going to be you. The only one who can push you through this and get you to where you want to go is you.

Even people who go on a monitored program need to realize that at the end of the day this is all about and for them. The professionals are not getting anything out of it, except maybe money and another client reference. It is their job, but this is your life, your wellbeing, and your quality of life.

Self-help books, trained and qualified professionals, support groups, and family can only get you to a certain point. It is like going up to the top of the tallest building fearing heights. Why go up there if you are unwilling to take that one small step that will allow you to see for miles around you? Until you are willing to try and take that step there really is no point in going up there. Just like intermittent fasting and clean eating, if you are unwilling to take that first step and commit, you are not going to get anywhere.

Doing all the groundwork to gear yourself up to start with fasting and a new diet is like taking that long ride up to the top of the building. You may think, "I will do it next time" or "I will start tomorrow". But what if next time or tomorrow is too late?

Procrastination is a person's worst enemy and leads to the inevitable if only statement. 'If only' does not help anyone and leads to depression, low self-esteem, and regret. But 'wow look at me now' energy leads to high spirits, high self-esteem, confidence-filled energy and vitality. It is taking that chance to step forward and trust that you will not fall only to be rewarded with breathtaking scenery and a feeling of triumph.

Can do and will do attitudes are the way to success. Losing weight and fasting are mostly a mindset, get yours in the correct set to achieve your goals.

Make yourself want to try new food groups, get excited about trying something new. Think about how you feel after a good scrub in the shower or day at the spa. How clean, shiny, and new you feel. When you go shopping for food or order from a restaurant or look at dinner menus think about feeling clean on the inside.

Mental Clarity

Fasting helps with mental clarity as it gives the body time to clean itself out and do a lot of reparative housework. Housework is hard to do when the body has to continually digest food from morning through to the evening.

Starting to fast, as with starting anything new, is hard and takes a lot of discipline as well as committed dedication. Most people who have trained their entire lives and stuck to healthy lifestyles may be able to make the adjustment to fasting more quickly.

But like dieting it is a mental transition. One of the best ways to make the transition is to start off with an activity that balances as well as centers a person. Some good examples of finding balance are meditation, the art of breathing, and exercises like yoga or tai chi.

Mindfulness Meditation

There have been studies that show meditation may be beneficial to one's mental and physical health. Mindfulness comes in when a person becomes aware of everything around them and is present in the moment without becoming stressed or overwhelmed.

Even though every human being on the planet has the ability to be mindful we do not all practice it on a daily basis. If you think of someone who is experienced in a trained discipline like martial arts. They learn to use their senses to be mindful of all those around them. They train their senses to become alert and can actually sense danger.

Animals in the wild use these senses every minute of their lives to stay alive. As apex predators and having been spoiled by not having to hunt or forage for our food, human beings' senses have been dulled. As a result, most of us have lost touch with more than just the world around us but our inner selves as well.

Mindful meditation is meant as a way to re-tune those senses and wake them up. Being mindful may actually rewire the physical structure of a person's brain. Research has shown that over time meditation creates some changes in the grey matter of the brain. In a control study group, participants of a meditation study reported they were less stressed, they felt better able to cope with their daily life after 27-hours of collective meditation over a period of time. (Holzel, Carmody, Vangel, Congleton, Yerramsetti, Gard, Lazar, 2011)

Meditation in itself is a journey we take into our minds. It is learning how to explore the fascinating system that is our body. Understanding its uniqueness, its likes and dislikes, and what it needs. It is a discovery of experiencing the full feeling of our senses, emotions, as well as our thoughts.

Mixing mindfulness in with meditation gives that journey another dimension and forces us to open up more than just what is within us. It helps us experience what is around us as well and how that affects us on a subconscious level.

Once you understand meditation, you will find that you can slip in and out of that state whenever or wherever. Even if it is just for a minute or two to quiet your mind and restore calm. It is within these moments where we can also put into practice mindfulness as we take that moment to concentrate on our breath and surroundings.

Mindful meditation helps a person achieve peace and calm within. It is a good place to start to take the next step towards fasting. It is also where you can reprogram yourself to accept the new lifestyle change and embrace the many benefits it is going to bring.

Fasting and meditation bring a great balance to a person's lifestyle. These practices have been used together for centuries. They have been used by various cultures to purify both the body and the soul. When used together they can become a powerful tool in understanding just how powerful the mind-body connection truly is.

Learning To Breathe

To breathe is done as a reflex, in fact, we are so used to this reflex we hardly pay attention to our breath. On average a person will take around 23,000 breaths without even realizing it. Well, unless there is a problem or an unappealing smell around us.

Buddhist monks are taught to be aware of their breath as it cultivates physical, mental, and emotional well-being. They use the breath to help them achieve mindfulness, balance and align their focus. Buddha teaches that to attain the Four Establishments of Mindfulness one must first be able to practice mindful breathing.

The four establishments of mindfulness are:

- Being mindful of our body.
- Being mindful of our mind and subconscious.
- Being mindful of our emotions, feelings, and sensations.
- Being mindful of the objects which are in our mind.

Learning to use our breath correctly to center and balance us to mindfulness helps to improve a person's concentration and thus their focus. By becoming aware of our breath, we allow it to flow more freely, we can use it to control stress, pain, and emotions. It can heighten our sensations and establish greater awareness within us and around us.

Learning to use our breath with mindful meditation is one more powerful tool to increase the benefits of intermittent fasting. It is also a way to help ready ourselves to accept and cope with intermittent fasting. Being able to breathe and control our breath also helps with our physical fitness, it can also lift any fog clouding the brain.

If you are feeling fatigued, irritated, or are running out of energy, straighten your diaphragm and practice your breathing. Once you are aware of your breathing, you can start realizing your breathing patterns. For instance, when some people get stressed, they tend to hold in their breath for longer periods of time. When you are anxious or angry, your breathing may become more rapid and your heart rate speeds up.

Knowing how to breathe to get your emotions and body in check is a good way to alleviate stress, anxiety, and lower your blood pressure too.

Movement

Mindfulness meditation and breathing can be combined with the gentle art of movement. You can try yoga which helps to strengthen your core, balance, and improves blood flow. It helps to cleanse your mind, body, and soul as energy flows through you.

Tai chi is another discipline that gently exercises the body, clears the mind, practices mindful breathing, and allows energy to flow through you. Tai chi is good for improving posture, improving physical balance, increasing muscle strength, and mobility. It is so gentle it can be practiced well into advanced years.

Putting It All Together

If you start off with one of the above techniques and stick to it. It will seem like a natural progression to the next stage which would be to start intermittent fasting. Once you start to feel the benefits of fasting, mindful meditation, breathing, and movement you will want to eat healthily.

Building yourself up for success is better done in stages than just jumping in feet first. You are establishing a new way of life one section at a time. Adapting and modifying one part of the process before moving onto the next process until you have reached your goal.

Chapter 6:
What You Need to Know

There are a few things that a person needs to know before diving in and proceeding with intermittent fasting. One of the first things is that it may be a good idea to have a general checkup and chat with your medical practitioner before you start fasting. A few blood workups or a complete physical can establish a baseline from which to begin. You will be able to figure out an ideal fasting plan as well as a suitable diet that includes any supplements, micronutrients, and macronutrients you may require.

Why the Intermittent Fasting Diet is More Than Just Weight Loss

The intermittent fasting diet is more than just a diet. It is a lifestyle choice. When you put the word diet on anything it automatically causes a mental block. That is a person's first stumbling block and one that can be removed easily enough. Rather think about intermittent fasting as making a lifestyle choice to improve your physical, mental, and overall health. The weight loss that may come with it, is an added bonus. It will also boost your self-esteem and energy levels which will in themselves greatly improve the quality of your life.

Intermittent fasting offers all the health benefits already discussed in this book along with learning self-control which leads to self-discipline. It offers mental clarity and puts you in tune with your body as you learn to differentiate between real hunger and that phantom hunger that demands satisfaction. Intermittent fasting makes you feel refreshed, clean and energized from the inside out. It is not a feeling you can gain from exercise, detoxing, or leading a healthy lifestyle it can only be felt after a bout of fasting.

You sleep better, heal better, feel better, have more energy, and as your mind is not foggy you are able to think on your feet. As a result, your stress levels decrease as anxiety starts to wane, and you feel more like a whole person again. But as with everything in life, it does come with warnings as we have stressed numerous times throughout the book. Intermittent fasting may not be for everyone and, depending on your health, you may need a modified version of one of the fasting methods.

What You Need to Know About Intermittent Fasting

Until you are well trained in intermittent fasting you should make yourself a schedule of your fasting days and times. The most straightforward intermittent fasting method to start on is the 5:2 method. In this method, you eat normally for 5 days of the week and then fast for the other 2 days. You will need to pick the two days of the week that will best suit you, making sure there is at least one to two days between fasting days.

During the two fasting days of the week, as a woman, you should consume no more than 500 calories a day. You can consume beverages that contain no calories as already discussed. Beverages like tea, coffee, and water with no added sweeteners. Water is always the best option as it makes you feel full and is an excellent source of hydration

Fasting Plan for 5:2 Combined With 12:12

When you are first starting out you may want to have a four-week cycle.

For instance:

Week 1

Fasting Days are Monday and Thursday. Fasting time is 12 hours with only non-caloric beverages and 12 hours where you can eat a maximum of 500 calories per day (two meals).

For Monday start fasting at 9 pm on Sunday night after you have had a good filling supper and stop fasting at 9 am Monday Morning until 9 pm on Monday night. Have an unsweetened coffee or tea for breakfast at 9 am, lunch to a total of 250 calories at 1 pm, and then supper at 7 or 8 pm of 250 calories. Tuesday morning you can start eating normally for the day.

For Thursday start fasting at 9 pm on Wednesday night after you have enjoyed a nice hearty supper. Follow the same fasting regiment as above and eat normally from Friday.

Week 2

Choose two different weekdays like Tuesday and Friday.

For Tuesday start fasting at 9 pm on Monday night after a hearty supper and follow the same method as Monday/Thursday above. Eat normally on Wednesday and Thursday for the day.

Friday you can start to fast at 9 pm on Thursday night once again after a good supper. Follow the same method as Monday, Thursday, and Tuesday above. You can start eating normally on Saturday morning again.

Week 3

Choose another two different days of the week like Wednesday and Saturday. Most people balk at having to fast on a Saturday, but it takes great discipline and you can always keep Sundays as your non-fasting day.

Wednesday you will start fasting at 9 pm on Tuesday night, following the same method as the days above, to start eating normally again on Thursday morning.

Saturday you will start fasting at 9 pm on Friday night. Follow the same method as the days above where you can start eating normally on Sunday morning.

Week 4

On week 4 you should not fast but instead eat normally every day then start the fasting week over the next week again.

Non-Fasting Days

As with the methods above, the days where you are not fasting you will eat a normal diet. Although there are no specific diet rules to follow when you are on eating days, or eating windows, it is highly recommended to follow a good, nutritious diet. After all, you want to reap the full benefits of this way of life, see results, and feel better. You may still reap some of the benefits if you eat what you like.

To make life even easier for you, find out what your recommended daily calorie intake is. This is determined by your height, bone structure, muscle mass, the way you carry your fat deposits, as well as your age and gender.

Once you have that you can find out what your weekly calorie intake should be.

For example, an average woman needs 2,000 calories a day to maintain a healthy weight, fasting days are 25% of the 2,000 calories (500 calories).

2,000 calories per day x 7 days = 14,000 calories a week

500 calories per day x 2 fasting days = 1,000 calories a week for fasting days

14,000 calories per week - 1,000 calories a week for fasting days = 13,000 calories a week

13,000 calories per week / 5 non-fasting days per week = 2,800 calories per non-fasting days

You should eat within your weekly calorie amount and not go over. It is better to try and keep your calories either at 14,000 calories per week and 2,000 calories per non-fasting days. To really boost your metabolism, try calorie cycling with your non-fasting days. Calories cycling is when you eat 2,000 calories one day, 1,000 calories another day, then 2,250 calories on another day, non-fasting days that is.

When calorie cycling you must not exceed your weekly calorie amount. If you start your calorie cycling on a Monday, then you only have until that Sunday night to eat your weekly amount. The following Monday your calories set back to 14,000 calories.

Choose a good diet or make healthy food choices if you are going to continue with your normal eating patterns. You do not have to make drastic changes but instead of reaching for a treat full of empty carbs reach for one that has some nutritional value. They are not loaded with anything artificial and taste just as good. Before you know it, you will have retrained your mind to rather opt for the healthier alternative to your favorite foods or beverages.

7-Day Intermittent Food Plan

One way to keep on a healthy diet is to plan your meals for the week ahead of time. That way you can get the shopping done more efficiently as you know exactly what you want to buy. It is also a great way to budget. You can prepare some meals in advance to save time, and you keep yourself on a healthy eating track.

Food Plan

The following 7-day meal plan is an example of what you can eat on your fasting days and non-fasting days. Remember to stay within your weekly calorie limit and go for the healthier choices. For instance, instead of taking full-fat vanilla ice cream, choose low-fat and sugar-free. Choose raw almonds instead of salted ones and so on.

Day 1 — Fasting Day 500 Calorie Allowance

9:00 AM Breakfast — 0 calories

A cup of unsweetened coffee or tea.

1:00 PM Lunch — 231 calories

1 small baked potato with ½ tsp butter and 2 tsp sour cream topped with ½ tsp chopped fresh chives.

Garden salad with ¼ cup of iceberg lettuce, 1 small celery stalk, 1 medium tomato, and drizzle with 1 tsp of balsamic vinegar.

8:00 PM Supper — 223 calories

¼ medium avocado, 1 tsp balsamic vinegar, and 1 slice of whole-wheat toast.

Add the same garden salad as above and add ¼ cucumber.

Day 2 — Non-Fasting Day 2 000 Calorie Allowance

9:00 AM Breakfast — 412 calories

2-egg omelet with 2 tbsp cheddar cheese, 1 tsp chopped spring onion, and 1 tbsp chopped button mushrooms.

1 slice of whole wheat toast with 1 tsp butter.

11:00 AM Snack — 166 calories

½ cup low-fat Greek yogurt, with 1 tsp organic honey, and ½ cup halved strawberries (fresh or frozen).

1:00 PM Lunch — 491 calories

6 shoots of grilled asparagus and 1 salmon fillet with lemon butter and dill sauce.

1 bowl of Caesar salad with dressing and croutons.

1 cup sugar-free butterscotch pudding.

3:00 PM Snack — 150 calories

2 tbsp feta cheese, ¼ cup of olives, 2 tbsp low-fat cottage cheese, 3 small breadsticks.

8:00 PM Supper — 698 calories

1 flame-grilled cheeseburger with a 1 cup of oven-baked fries with low-sodium salt to taste.

1 cup fat-free vanilla ice cream with ½ cup blueberries (fresh or frozen) and ½ cup raspberries (fresh or frozen).

10:00 PM Snack — 66 calories

½ cup of blackberries and 5 raw almonds.

Day 3 — Non-Fasting Day 2 000 Calorie Allowance

9:00 AM Breakfast — 492 calories

1 cup of organic rolled oats cooked, add ¼ cup unsweetened almond milk, 1 sliced banana, ¼ cup mixed berries (frozen or fresh), 3 tsp organic honey, and 2 tbsp raw almond slices.

11:00 AM Snack — 128 calories

½ cup low-fat plain chunky cottage cheese with 2 tsp organic honey, 2 tbsp blackberries, 2 tbsp raspberries, and 1 tbsp raw cashew nuts. The berries can be either fresh or frozen and the cashews should be unsalted.

1:00 PM Lunch — 393 calories

2 slices whole wheat bread, 2 tsp butter, 2 slices of turkey, 2 tbsp shredded cheddar cheese, 1 tsp low-fat mayonnaise, ¼ sliced tomato, 2 lettuce leaves, and 2 tsp alfalfa sprouts. Make a delicious filling sandwich.

Slice up ¼ apple, 5 grapes, 2 tbsp low-fat Greek yogurt, 1 tsp organic honey, ¼ tsp ground cinnamon, and ¼ tsp cayenne pepper for extra zing (optional). Mix together in a dessert bowl for a treat after your sandwich.

3:00 PM Snack — 173 calories

2 plain, no salt added rice cakes, 2 tbsp plain low-fat cream cheese, 1 tsp organic honey, and ¼ tsp ground cinnamon. Spread a bit of cream cheese on each rice cake, drizzle with a bit of the honey and add a dash of ground cinnamon on top.

8:00 PM Supper — 692 calories

1 lean grilled chicken breast (spiced as you require and cut into chunks), ¼ cup cooked wild rice, ¼ tsp ground ginger, ¼ tsp ground cinnamon, ¼ cup cooked garden peas, 3 tbsp diced spring onions, and 1 tbsp low-fat mayonnaise. Serve the chicken and rice warm, add the rest of the ingredients after you have mixed up the rice and chicken in a dinner bowl.

1 cup fat-free vanilla ice cream with ½ cup fresh, halved strawberries, 1 diced kiwi, and ½ cup diced fresh mango.

Drizzle with 1 tsp organic honey and sprinkle with all-spice as well as chopped raw cashews.

10:00 PM Snack — 139 calories

20 raw almonds.

Day 4 — Fasting Day 500 Calorie Allowance

9:00 AM Breakfast — 0 calories

A cup of unsweetened coffee or tea.

1:00 PM Lunch — 269 calories

2 large bell peppers (cut in half), 3 tbsp cooked wild rice, 1 tsp capers, ½ oz lean grilled chicken breasts shredded, and 2 tsp reduced-fat mayonnaise. Divide filling and stuff evenly between each bell pepper half.

8:00 PM Supper — 224 calories

1 grilled sole fillet with 1 tsp garlic butter.

Garden salad with 1 cup of iceberg lettuce, 1 medium tomato chopped, ¼ cucumber, 1 tbsp spring onions, ½ cup button mushrooms, 2 tbsp yellow bell pepper, and 1 tbsp organic balsamic vinegar.

Day 5 — Non-Fasting Day 2 000 Calorie Allowance

9:00 AM Breakfast — 528 calories

2 eggs scrambled with 2 tbsp shredded cheddar cheese, 2 tbsp shredded mozzarella cheese, and 1 tsp chopped spring onion.

2 slice of whole wheat toast with 1 tsp butter

1 medium apple

11:00 AM Snack — 173 calories

¼ cup regular trail mix

1:00 PM Lunch — 523 calories

1 low-carb whole wheat tortilla stuffed with shredded lettuce, ½ chopped tomato, 4 cooked and crumbled pieces of bacon, ¼ chopped avocado, 2 chopped pickles, 1 tbsp low-fat mayonnaise.

1 medium-sized peach

3:00 PM Snack — 118 calories

Mixed berry smoothie, 2 tbsp blueberries, 2 tbsp blackberries, 2 tbsp raspberries, ¼ cup organic low-fat unsweetened almond milk, and 4 tbsp low-fat Greek yogurt.

8:00 PM Supper — 683 calories

1 large whole wheat tortilla, spread the base with 2 tsp organic unsweetened tomato paste, top with 4 tbsp shredded mozzarella cheese, top with 1 cup cooked shredded chicken breast, ½ thinly sliced tomato. Then top with ½ tsp capers, 1 tbsp pitted black olives, drizzle with 2 tbsp fruit chutney, and last sprinkle 4 tbsp shredded cheddar cheese over the top. Pop the tortilla pizza into a preheated oven and cook for around 18 to 20 minutes or until brown and the ingredients are cooked.

1 large banana sliced lengthwise, ¼ cup fat-free vanilla ice cream, ¼ mixed berries fresh or frozen, 1 large plum cut into chunks, ½ pear cut into chunks, and 1 tbsp unsweetened desiccated coconut. Make the ingredients into a banana boat and top with the desiccated coconut.

10:00 PM Snack — 150 calories

4 pieces of dark chocolate.

Day 6 — Non-Fasting Day 2 000 Calorie Allowance

9:00 AM Breakfast — 348 calories

In a dessert bowl or parfait glass add 4 tbsp organic sugar-free granola, top with 5 tbsp fat-free strawberry yogurt, top with 1 tbsp blackberries, 1 tbsp raspberries, 1 tbsp blueberries. Then top with 4 tbsp fat-free plain Greek yogurt, drizzle over 1 tsp organic, honey, sprinkle 1 tsp of toasted almond flakes, 1 tsp chia seeds, and 1 tsp unsweetened desiccated coconut.

11:00 AM Snack — 183 calories

1 peanut butter protein bar

2 small apricots

1:00 PM Lunch — 413 calories

1 bowl of chicken Caesar salad with dressing and croutons

1 large banana

1 cup of grapes

3:00 PM Snack — 184 calories

¼ cup of olives

½ cup of fresh cauliflower divided into florets

½ cup carrots cut into sticks

½ cup cucumber cut into sticks

¼ cup tzatziki

8:00 PM Supper — 653 calories

1 roasted chicken breast, 4 roast potatoes, ½ cup cooked corn, ½ cup cooked carrots, and ½ cup cooked peas

1 cup fat-free vanilla ice cream topped with 2 tsp organic cocoa powder, 2 tsp organic honey, and 1 tbsp raw unsalted cashews.

10:00 PM Snack — 150 calories

4 pieces of dark chocolate.

Day 7 — Non-Fasting Day 2 000 Calorie Allowance

9:00 AM Breakfast — 399 calories

1 chopped apple, 1 chopped plum, ¼ papaya chopped, 1 banana sliced, ¼ cup fresh halved strawberries, ¼ cup blueberries, 1 tsp sunflower seeds, and 2 tbsp low-fat vanilla Greek yogurt.

1 glass unsweetened organic light coconut milk.

11:00 AM Snack — 150 calories

4 pieces of dark chocolate.

1:00 PM Lunch — 657 calories

1 bowl of chicken soup with 2 slices of whole wheat toast and 2 tsp butter.

1 small green salad.

1 cup sugar-free butterscotch pudding with ½ cup of fat-free vanilla ice cream.

3:00 PM Snack — 228 calories

3 graham crackers with 1 tbsp Nutella.

8:00 PM Supper — 795 calories

1 grilled chicken burger with a 1 cup of oven-baked fries with low-sodium salt to taste.

1 small green salad.

1 slice of cheesecake, 1 tbsp low-fat unsweetened whipped cream, and 1 tsp macadamia nuts.

10:00 PM Snack 104 calories

½ cup of blackberries, ½ cup of raspberries, and ¼ of blueberries.

7-Day Food Plan Calorie Summary

Day 1 (fasting day) = 454 calories in total which is 46 calories less than the daily allowance.

Day 2 (normal eating day) = 1 983 calories in total which is 17 calories less than the daily allowance.

Day 3 (normal eating day) = 2 017 calories in total which is 17 calories more than the daily allowance.

Day 4 (fasting day) = 493 calories in total which is 7 calories less than the daily allowance.

Day 5 (normal eating day) = 2 175 calories in total which is 175 calories more than the daily allowance.

Day 6 (normal eating day) = 1 931 calories in total which is 69 calories less than the daily allowance.

Day 7 (normal eating day) = 2 333 calories in total which is 333 calories more than the daily allowance.

Total calories for the week = 11 386 calories which is 2614 calories less than the weekly total.

As you can see by the meal plan that you can eat great meals, with dessert and still come in well under the recommended calorie intake for the week. All you have to do is make healthier food choices when shopping, going out to eat, or at a dinner party.

Chapter 7:
Ideas for Breakfast, Lunch, and Supper

Eating healthy greatly complements your new fasting lifestyle. But you also have to ensure that you are getting enough nutrition in your diets as well.

Eating Nutritiously for Women Aged 50 and Over

As a woman, your body has certain nutrient needs that must be fulfilled to maintain good health. You can get a good source of these vitamins and minerals through supplements, but nothing beats the more natural way through food sources.

A lot of women tend to fall short of getting in their daily nutritional requirements. Getting in the correct nutritional requirements can also improve your energy levels, mood, and help control weight gain. As your body ages, you need to help keep it functioning correctly with the correct nutrition. It can also help you through menopause and beyond to ensure you have a good quality of life.

When you are fasting, it is really important to get in as much of your daily recommended nutrients as possible. These help the body to produce hormones and energy, keep the skin healthy, promote healthy teeth, hair, nails, and bones.

The RDA (recommended daily allowance) of the vital nutrients for women 50 and over are:

Calcium - 1,200 mg per day

Calcium is needed for strong bones and healthy teeth. It also aids in regulating the heartbeat and a deficiency of it affects your teeth, bones, and mood. Not getting enough calcium can lead to osteoporosis. This is because the body will start to take calcium from the bones to aid normal cell function.

Foods that are high in calcium include:

- Low-fat, plain Greek yogurt
- Full-cream milk, non-fat milk, 2% milk, or reduced-fat milk (find a variety fortified with vitamin D).
- Cheeses: cheddar, mozzarella, cream cheese, feta, parmesan, and cottage cheese
- Tofu that states it is made with calcium sulfate
- Nut milk
- Soy milk
- Kale, broccoli, Chinese cabbage, and turnips
- Salmon, shrimp, and sardines
- Oranges and figs
- Fortified cereals
- Baked beans or most canned beans

Iron - 8 mg per day

Iron is an important nutrient the body needs to maintain healthy hair, skin, nails, and hemoglobin. Hemoglobin is the compound that oxygenates the blood. A deficiency of iron can cause anemia which can cause a person to feel weak and lethargic.

Foods that are high in iron include:

- Raisins
- Bell peppers
- Leafy green vegetables like spinach
- Eggs (boiled)

- Cashew nuts
- Potatoes
- Broccoli, peas, and green beans
- Tuna, oysters, sardines, and muscles
- Turkey and chicken
- Liver
- Beef
- Kidney beans, white beans, lentils, and chickpeas
- Tomatoes
- Bread
- Tofu
- Nuts and seeds
- Some dried fruit
- Breakfast cereals
- Dark chocolate

Magnesium - 400 mg per day

Magnesium is a nutrient needed to help keep bones and teeth healthy. It also aids in ensuring that your nervous systems and muscles work correctly. Magnesium is needed to support proper insulin levels as well as heart health.

Foods that are high in magnesium include:

- Avocado
- Dark chocolate
- Nuts and seeds
- Most fruit especially raspberries, bananas and figs
- Chickpeas, kidney beans, baked beans, and black beans
- Peas, broccoli, cabbage, green beans, asparagus, and artichokes
- Tuna, mackerel, salmon, and sardines
- Bread, oats, and brown rice
- Cacao (raw organic)

- Tofu
- Leafy green vegetables like kale, spinach, and lettuce

Vitamin A - 700 mcg per day

Vitamin A is a multifunctional vitamin that plays an important role in keeping the internal organs, kidney, lungs, and heart working as they should. It also supports the immune system, reproduction system, and eyesight.

Foods that are high in vitamin A include:

- Liver
- Cod liver oil
- Tuna, mackerel, trout, and salmon
- Butter
- Cheese, especially goat cheese
- Boiled egg
- Sweet potato, butternut squash, and carrots
- Spinach, broccoli, bell pepper, and lettuce
- Melons and grapefruit

Vitamin C - 75 mg per day

Vitamin C is another vitamin that plays a crucial part in many operations within the body. It aids the immune system, repairs cell tissue, is vital for growth and normal development. It helps the body absorb iron, and sees to the care of bones, teeth, and muscles. It plays an important part in skin health as it helps with the creation of collagen as well as the healing of wounds.

Foods that are high in vitamin C include:

- Oranges
- Clementines
- Grapefruit
- Kiwis

- Pineapple
- Apricots
- Mangos
- Guava
- Strawberries
- Papaya
- Bell peppers
- Kale
- Brussel Sprouts
- Broccoli
- Cauliflower
- Yellow melons
- Chilis

Vitamin B-6 - 1.5 mg per day

The B vitamins work together to help with the metabolism, growth, liver function, and the creation of blood cells. Vitamin B-6 is used in the production of the sleep hormone, melatonin.

Foods that are high in vitamin B-6 include:

- Peanuts
- Eggs
- Fish
- Poultry
- Pork
- Bread
- Wholegrain cereals
- Fortified cereals
- Potatoes
- Milk
- Vegetables
- Soya beans

Vitamin B-9 (Folate) - 400 mcg per day

The B vitamins work together and with other nutrients to create red blood cells. Folate is also an important vitamin that ensures iron is properly absorbed and used in the body. Vitamin B-9 is used to aid in regulating the amino acid homocysteine blood levels.

Foods that are high in vitamin B-9 include:

- Seafood
- Eggs
- Most fresh fruit
- Most fresh fruit juices
- Liver
- Peanuts
- Beans
- Whole grains
- Sunflower seeds
- Broccoli
- Turnip greens
- Asparagus
- Spinach
- Brussel sprouts
- Lettuce
- Green beans

Vitamin B-12 - 2.4 mcg per day

Vitamin B-12 helps to prevent anemia as it aids the body in properly absorbing and utilizing iron. It helps in the production of DNA and regulates the blood cells and the nervous system.

Foods that are high in vitamin B-12 include:

- Kidneys
- Liver

- Beef
- Other edible animal organs
- Sardines, tuna, trout, herring, and salmon
- Clams, shrimp, mussels, crab, and oysters
- Fortified dairy products
- Eggs
- Ham and pork
- Chicken and turkey
- Plain Greek yogurt
- Cottage, cream cheese, ricotta and mozzarella cheese
- Nutritional yeast

Vitamin D - 15 mg per day

One of the main functions of vitamin D is helping the body to absorb calcium to ensure healthy bones and teeth. It also supports the immune system, promotes good skin health, may reduce depression, and it can increase weight loss.

Foods that are high in vitamin D include:

- Some nuts and seeds contain vitamin D
- Beef liver
- Egg yolk
- Tuna, salmon, and mackerel
- Fortified dairy products
- Fortified cereals

Vitamin E — 15 mcg per day

Vitamin E is like the soldier nutrient of the body. It is used to help fight off harmful bacteria, protects cells against damage, it is an antioxidant, and it boosts the immune system. Vitamin E is also vital for firmer, younger-looking skin.

Foods that are high in vitamin E include:

- Almonds

- Pine nuts
- Peanuts
- Seeds like sunflower seeds
- Spinach
- Broccoli
- Butternut squash
- Avocado
- Kiwi
- Mangos
- Shrimp
- Lobster
- Trout, salmon, and cod
- Goose
- Olive oil

Vitamin K - 90 mcg per day

Vitamin K is an important nutrient that helps with bone metabolism and controls calcium levels in the blood. It is also a very important agent that helps in the production of prothrombin which is a protein used in blood clotting.

Foods that are high in vitamin K include:

- Swiss chard
- Mustard greens
- Kale
- Spinach and broccoli
- Liver
- Prunes
- Kiwi
- Hard cheeses
- Avocado
- Green peas
- Cabbage
- Broccoli

Healthy Eating Ideas

While fasting you should try to eat breakfast later in the day if you are fasting through the night.

If you have chosen the fasting meal plan that allows a person to consume a limited number of calories per day, try to eat only two meals a day — lunch and supper. But if you must eat breakfast then make it a smaller one, take no more than 50 calories from lunch and 70 from dinner. It is better to keep the evening meal lighter than your afternoon one as you need the energy from lunch to get you through the entire day.

Fasting Plan Without Calorie Restriction

Drink a lot of water which may be infused with mint. Mint keeps you alert and gives the water a nice flavor, but you cannot put anything to sweeten it in the water.

Drink tea or coffee with no sweeteners, sugar, cream, or flavors. You may put a dash of cayenne pepper in the drink to give it a kick and help burn calories.

Fasting Plan With Calorie Restriction

Fasting day with calorie-restrictive eating windows is based on 500 calories a day.

The breakdown for 500 calories fasting day restriction would be:

With a small breakfast

- Breakfast = 130 calories
- Lunch = 200 calories
- Dinner = 170 calories

Lunch and dinner only

- Breakfast = 0 calories

- Lunch = 250 calories
- Dinner = 250 calories

Normal Eating (Non-Fasting) Days or Eating Window Food Ideas

Non-fasting day food ideas are based on an average of 2,000 calories a day. If you are wanting to lose weight you should look at cutting that down to around 1,500 calories a day.

The breakdown for normal day eating at 2,000 calories a day (14,000 calories per week) would be:

- Breakfast = 500 calories
- Mid-morning snack = 200 calories
- Lunch = 500 calories
- Mid-afternoon snack = 200 calories
- Dinner = 500 calories
- Light before bed snack = 100 calories

Always drink a glass of warm water before going to sleep. Warm water will help stave off night cramps, relieve pain, and helps to rid the body of unwanted toxins. This is because warm water is great for circulation. It will also keep you hydrated during the long hours of the night which in turn will help you have a good quality night's rest.

Healthy Breakfast Ideas

The following are a few quick and simple healthy breakfast ideas to help kick start your morning.

Fasting Without Limited Calories

This is usually done during the evening and into mid-morning the following day. If it does span a day there are non-fasting windows where a person can eat normally. See the non-fasting healthy ideas for normal eating day breakfast ideas.

Fasting With Limited Calories (100 to 130 Calories)

The following recipes are 130 calories and under.

Blueberry Mango Yogurt - 97 Calories

- 1 small mango chopped
- 1 oz blueberries (fresh or frozen)
- 4 tbsp non-fat plain Greek yogurt
- dash of ground cinnamon

Spoon the yogurt into a parfait glass or dessert bowl, add the chopped mango and blueberries. Add a dash of cinnamon for taste and to add a bit of sweetness.

Egg White Mushroom Scramble - 93 Calories

- 3 tbsp fresh button mushrooms chopped
- 3 fresh egg whites
- 1 tsp coconut oil to cook with
- low-sodium salt and black pepper to taste

Heat the coconut oil in a skillet over medium heat. Add the egg whites and mushrooms stir into a scramble then serve hot.

Cold Watermelon, Grapefruit, Kiwi, and Pomegranate Cup - 100 Calories

- 1 tbsp pomegranate seeds
- ½ small chopped kiwi fruit

- ½ small grapefruit
- ¼ cup iced, cubed fresh watermelon

Freeze the watermelon the night before. Add all the chopped fruit to a cereal or dessert bowl and enjoy a fresh fruit salad for breakfast.

Almonds, Banana, and Honey - 129 Calories

- 1 small banana sliced
- 1 tbsp organic coconut flakes
- 1 tsp organic honey

Slice the banana and add it to a cereal or dessert bowl. Drizzle with organic honey, sprinkle over the coconut flakes and enjoy.

Mixed Berry Coconut Smoothie - 121 Calories

- 3 tbsp blueberries
- 3 tbsp raspberries
- 3 tbsp blackberries
- 2 tsp shredded unsweetened coconut shreds
- ¼ cup unsweetened coconut water
- ½ cup still mineral water
- 1 tsp organic honey
- dash of cinnamon to taste

Add all the ingredients into a blender. Blend until the smoothie is thick and smooth. Add to a glass and drink or pack it in a container to take with you.

Healthy Breakfast Ideas for Normal Eating Days (500 Calories and Under)

These easy breakfast recipes are filled with nutrients and are only 500 calories or less.

Boiled Egg, Avocado, and Red Radish, Rocket Breakfast Salad - 471 Calories

- ½ avocado cubed
- ¼ cucumber sliced
- ¼ cup of rocket
- ¼ cup baby spinach leaves
- 3 large radishes sliced into rounds
- 2 hard-boiled eggs, halved
- 4 tbsp fat-free chunky cottage cheese
- low-sodium salt and black pepper to taste
- 1 slice wholewheat toast
- 1 tsp low-fat unsalted butter
- 1 tbsp balsamic vinegar

Add all the fresh ingredients to a salad bowl, toss, and drizzle with balsamic vinegar, add low-sodium salt and black pepper to taste. Halve the hard-boiled eggs and place them on top of the salad. Spread the whole wheat toast with the teaspoon of butter and serve with the salad.

Spicy Mashed Sardines Mixed with Feta and Pickles on Whole Wheat Toast - 382 Calories

- 5 tbsp sardines, drained and mashed
- 2 slices of whole wheat toast
- 1 tbsp feta cheese
- 2 diced pickles
- 2 tsp butter
- dash of cayenne pepper to taste and add a zing

Mash the sardines with the feta and diced pickles add a dash of cayenne pepper for zing. Toast two slices of whole wheat bread and spread each one with the butter. Divide the sardines and spread onto each slice of toast to enjoy.

Chocolate, Mixed Berry, Banana, Apricot, and Oats Breakfast Smoothie - 243 Calories

- 4 tbsp rolled oats
- 5 tbsp dried apricots
- 2 tbsp raspberries
- 2 tbsp blackberries
- ¼ cup chopped strawberries
- ½ small banana chopped
- 2 tsp organic honey
- ¼ unsweetened coconut water
- ¼ cup filtered water
- 2 tsp fresh chopped mint
- 1 tsp raw organic cocoa

Blend all the ingredients together until the smoothie is thick and smooth. Add to a glass and drink or pack it in a container to take with you.

Tuna, Capers, Rocket, and Feta Omelet - 482 Calories

- 3 fresh eggs
- 4 tbsp canned tuna in water without added salt
- 2 tbsp feta cheese
- 4 tbsp chopped rocket
- 2 tbsp baby spinach leaves
- 1 tsp capers
- 1 slice whole wheat toast
- 1 tsp butter
- 1 tsp coconut oil cook with
- black pepper to taste

Scramble the eggs in a bowl. Heat the coconut oil in an omelet pan. Add the egg until it is almost completely cooked through. Add the tuna, feta, chopped rocket, baby spinach leaves, and capers to the one half of the egg mixture. Flip the free half over the ingredients to form an omelet fold. Cook on both sides for 1 to 2 minutes until the omelet is cooked through.

Toast the whole wheat bread and use the butter to spread it. Cut it into triangle halves and serve it with the hot omelet.

Banana, Pomegranate Granola - 459 Calories

- 4 tbsp pomegranate seeds
- 1 large banana sliced
- 1 cup organic unsweetened granola
- 2 tsp organic honey
- 4 tbsp vanilla low-fat Greek yogurt
- 1 tbsp sunflower seeds
- 1 tbsp shredded unsweetened coconut

Place the granola in a cereal bowl. Top with the Greek yogurt and sliced banana. Drizzle the honey over the granola and banana. Top with pomegranate seeds, sunflower seeds, and shredded coconut.

Healthy Lunch Ideas

Lunch is an important meal as it is the one that staves off the mid-morning hunger and gets you through the rest of the day. If you are going to eat a big meal, this would be a better time of the day to eat it. As you have to get through the next half of the day until supper you will be more likely to burn off most of the meal.

Fasting Without Limited Calories

This is usually done during the evening and into mid-morning the following day. This means that your normal eating window would start at around 11 am. See the non-fasting healthy ideas for normal eating day lunch ideas. Try and cut down on the calories in order to help keep your system balanced. Instead of wolfing down a large amount of food because you have just come off a fast, drink a glass or two of water before eating. This will make you feel full and then go about preparing your meal.

Fasting With Limited Calories (200 to 250 Calories)

The following lunches will go down well on fasting days with limited calories as they are all 250 calories and under.

Beets, Ginger, Spring Onion With Grilled Hake - 127 Calories

- 1 grilled hake steak
- ¼ cup shredded raw beets
- 2 tbsp shredded fresh ginger root
- 3 spring onions chopped
- 1 tsp chili spice
- low-sodium salt and black pepper to taste

Preheat the grill. Prepare the hake steak with low-sodium salt, black pepper, and chili spice. Place in the grill and cook until the steak is almost done, about 10 to 15 minutes. Turn the steak halfway through cooking to cook evenly. Top with shredded ginger root and spring onion. Place the dish back into the grill for another 5 to 8 minutes. Remove from the grill, dish up onto a plate and top with fresh beets.

Golden Chocolate Avocado Smoothie - 171 Calories

- ¼ chopped avocado
- ¼ small chopped banana
- 1 cup of filtered water
- ½ cup of ice cubes
- 1 tsp turmeric

- 1 tsp raw organic cocoa
- 1 tsp vanilla extract

Add all the ingredients into the blender. Blend until the smoothie is thick and smooth.

Chicken and Avocado in a Kale Wrap - 223 Calories

- ¼ avocado sliced
- ¼ cup shredded grilled chicken breast
- 2 large kale leaves
- 1 tbsp smooth cottage cheese
- low-sodium salt and black pepper to taste

Mix the salt and pepper with the cottage cheese. Mix the shredded chicken and avocado into the cottage cheese mix. Wash and pat the kale leaves dry then stack them on top of each other. Add the shredded chicken, avocado, and cottage cheese into the middle of the top kale leaf. Fold the leaf into a wrap over the mixture and enjoy. You can make three small wraps if you prefer.

Chicken Liver Stuffed Zucchini Boats - 198 Calories

- 1 large zucchini
- 4 tbsp cooked chicken livers
- 2 tbsp parmesan cheese
- ¼ cup mixed salad leaves
- 1 tsp pine nuts
- ¼ cherry tomatoes halved
- 1 tbsp feta cheese
- 2 tbsp pomegranate seeds
- 3 tsp balsamic vinegar
- low-sodium salt and black pepper to taste

Preheat the grill. Halve the zucchini cutting longways into two boats. Cut out a hollow (do not go right through the zucchini) in the middle of each boat. Put the cut-out zucchini flesh aside. Add the cooked chicken livers to the middle of the zucchini, dividing them evenly between the halves. Sprinkle parmesan over the top of the chicken livers, flavor with salt, and pepper. Place the zucchini boats into the grill for 8 to 10 minutes until cooked.

While the zucchini is cooking add the rest of the ingredients into a salad bowl, toss, and drizzle with balsamic vinegar. Add the extra zucchini cut out from the middle of the boat to the salad (chop into cubes). Flavor with salt and pepper to taste. When the zucchini boats are done serve with the salad.

Eggplant Jalapeno and Prawn Pizza Slices— 219 Calories

- 1 large eggplant
- 2 tsp jalapeno peppers
- 6 cleaned, grilled king prawns
- 1 tbsp organic unsweetened tomato paste
- 1 tbsp shredded mozzarella cheese
- 1 tbsp parmesan cheese

Preheat the oven to 340°F. Peel the eggplant and slice long ways into slices (not too thin). Spread tomato paste on one side of each slice. Top the tomato paste with shredded mozzarella. Chop the prawns into bits and place them on top of the tomato paste along with the jalapeno peppers. Sprinkle a good coating of parmesan over each pizza slice. Place on a prepared baking tray and put into the oven to bake until cooked.

Healthy Lunch Ideas for Normal Eating Days (500 Calories and Under)

Tuna and Chunky Cottage Cheese Baked Potato with a Green Salad - 383 Calories

- 1 can tuna in water without salt drained
- 2 tbsp chunky fat-free plain cottage cheese
- 1 large Idaho baking potato
- ¼ cup mixed salad leaves
- ¼ cucumber diced
- ¼ green bell pepper diced
- 2 tbsp pumpkin seeds
- 2 tsp fresh basil
- 3 tsp organic balsamic vinegar
- low-sodium salt and black pepper to taste

Add salt and pepper to the cottage cheese, mix in the tuna. Bake the potato and scoop out the middle and mix with the tuna mixture. Add the tuna mixture to the middle of the baked potato. Toss the salad ingredients (salad leaves, cucumber, bell pepper, pumpkin seeds, and fresh basil). Add salt and pepper to taste, drizzle with balsamic vinegar and serve with the baked potato.

Muscles, Lettuce, Capers, and Tomato Pita - 423 Calories

- 1 can of muscles, drained
- ¼ cup fresh shredded lettuce
- 1 whole wheat pita
- 1 tsp capers
- ½ large tomato diced
- 4 spring onions chopped
- ¼ cucumber diced
- 4 tsp smooth cottage cheese

- 1 tsp Dijon mustard
- ¼ tsp cayenne pepper

Mix together the cottage cheese, Dijon mustard, and cayenne pepper. Slice the top of the pita open and toast it until golden brown. In a bowl toss together the muscles, lettuce, capers, tomatoes, onions, and cucumber. Mix in the mayonnaise and Dijon mustard mix. Stuff the pita pocket with muscle mixture and enjoy it.

Toasted Chicken and Hot English Mustard Mayo Sandwich - 464 Calories

- 2 slices of whole wheat bread
- ½ cup of shredded grilled chicken breast
- 1 tbsp low-fat mayonnaise
- 1 tsp hot English mustard
- 1 cup of oven chips
- 2 tsp unsalted butter

Cook the oven chips and spice with Cajun spice if desired. Mix together the low-fat mayonnaise and hot English mustard. Add the shredded grilled chicken to the mayonnaise and mustard mix. Use the unsalted butter to butter the bread. Place the chicken on one slice of the bread, cover with the other slice and grill the sandwich until it is toasted.

Tuna, Prawn, Crab, and Lobster Salad - 429 Calories

- 6 king prawns cleaned and grilled
- 4 tbsp fresh cooked crab meat
- 4 tbsp fresh cooked lobster meat
- 1 tsp capers
- 1 tsp jalapeno peppers
- 2 tsp sliced olives
- ¼ cup mixed salad leaves

- 2 tbsp feta
- ½ avocado diced
- 1 tbsp sesame seeds
- 3 tbsp low-fat mayonnaise
- 2 tsp Dijon mustard
- 1 tsp organic balsamic vinegar
- 1 tsp tomato ketchup
- 1 tsp organic honey

In a small mixing bowl mix together the low-fat mayonnaise, Dijon mustard, ketchup, honey, and balsamic vinegar. In a salad bowl, toss together the salad ingredients including the seafood. Drizzle with the mustard salad dressing and enjoy.

Grilled Portobello Mushrooms with Feta Cheese and Avocado Bun - 500 Calories

- 1 large portobello mushroom
- 1 tbsp feta cheese
- 1 large avocado
- 1 cup tortilla chips
- 2 tsp sliced olives
- low-sodium salt and pepper to taste

Cut the stalk from the portobello mushroom and place it on a grilling dish with the stalk side up. Add some garlic flakes, low-sodium salt, and crumble feta cheese over the mushrooms. Place it on the grill and cook it until it starts to get soft and the feta has melted. Peel and cut the avocado in half longwise. Take out the pip, place the mushroom on the one half of the avocado. Cover the mushroom with the other half of the avocado making an avocado burger. Sever with 1 cup of tortilla chips and spice as desired.

Healthy Dinner Ideas

Dinner should be a hearty meal, especially if you are going to be fasting the next day or through the nighttime into the next day. Try to eat earlier in the evening to avoid going to bed and a full stomach as this will be hard to digest and may give your problems sleeping.

Fasting Without Limited Calories

Depending on your eating window this will probably be your second meal of the day during a fasting period. See the non-fasting healthy ideas for normal eating day dinner ideas. Once again try to control your portion sizes and gradually cut them down. Rather have a larger lunch than a larger dinner.

Try to eat before 7:30 pm in the evening.

Fasting With Limited Calories (170 to 250 Calories)

The following are deliciously healthy dinner meals that offer optimum nutrition for under 250 calories.

Ham and Cottage Cheese Chickpea Burger - 250 Calories

- 1 whole wheat burger bun
- 1 tbsp chopped cooked ham
- 2 tsp fat-free cottage cheese
- 1/4 cup mashed chickpeas
- 2 lettuce leaves
- ¼ tsp hot sauce

Drain and mash the chickpeas. Add the cottage cheese, hot sauce, and ham to the chickpea mixture. Pat the chickpea mixture into a burger patty shape. Grill for 8 to 10 minutes or until the chickpea patty has heated through. Halve the burger bun, place a lettuce leaf on each half. Put the chickpea patty on the bottom half, close the two halves and enjoy your burger.

Grilled Tuna on One Potato Mash - 239 Calories

- 1 Idaho potato, boiled, and mashed
- 1 grilled tuna steak
- 1 cup of baby spinach leaves
- 1 tsp pine nuts
- 1 tbsp feta cheese
- 1 tsp sunflower seeds
- 1 tsp raw chopped cashew nuts
- 2 tsp organic balsamic vinegar

Grill the tuna, seasoned with low-sodium salt and black pepper to taste. Boil and mash the Idaho potato. Toss the spinach leaves, pine nuts, sunflower seeds, cashews and feta in a salad bowl then drizzle with balsamic vinegar. Serve the tuna on top of the mash with the green salad on the side.

Vegetable and 3 Cheese Tart - 215 Calories per serving

- ½ eggplant
- 3 courgettes
- ½ red bell pepper
- ½ cup baby spinach leaves
- 2 tbsp olive slices
- 1 tbsp jalapeno peppers
- 1 roll of puff pastry
- 4 tbsp feta cheese
- 4 tbsp fat-free cottage cheese
- 2 tbsp parmesan cheese

This makes three servings.

Preheat the oven to 300°F. Prepare a baking tray with cooking spray. Roll out the filo pastry and place it in a pie shape at the bottom of the baking tray. Place the pastry into the oven until it starts to get brown. Cook the vegetables in a skillet with coconut oil over medium heat. When cooked, mix in the cream cheese and place them in the pie crust. Mix in olive slices and crumble feta over the vegetable mix. Sprinkle with parmesan cheese and place the pie back in the oven for another 8 to 10 minutes until the cheese has melted in. Remove from the oven and serve.

Asparagus, Green Bean, and Poached Egg Salad - 218 Calories

- 5 fresh grilled asparagus spears
- 1 cup grilled green beans
- 2 poached egg
- ½ cup baby spinach leaves
- ¼ cup rocket
- 4 tsp Dijon mustard

Lay a bed of baby spinach leaves mixed with rocket leaves. Place the grilled asparagus and beans onto the mixed leaves. Place the warm poached egg on the top, drizzle with Dijon mustard and enjoy.

Grilled Turkey Breast with Boiled Garlic and Ginger Butter Baby Potatoes - 250 Calories

- 4 washed and boiled baby potatoes
- ½ grilled turkey breast cut into slices
- 1 tsp grated fresh ginger root
- 1 tsp organic crushed garlic
- 3 tsp unsalted butter
- low-sodium salt and black pepper to taste

Place the hot grilled and sliced turkey breast on a plate with the boiled baby potatoes. In a pot melt the butter with the grated ginger root and garlic. When the butter is cooked, pour the mixture over the baby potatoes and serve. You can add some mixed salad leaves if you wish.

Dinner Ideas for Normal Eating Days (500 Calories and Under)

The following dinner ideas are quick and easy to make, are under 500 calories and high in healthy nutrition.

Bison Burger with Cajun Oven Baked Potato Wedges and Sour Cream - 500 Calories

- 1 bison burger patty
- 1 whole wheat bun
- 1 tbsp Dijon mustard
- 1 large pickle, thinly sliced
- 1 large washed lettuce leaf
- 1 slice of a large tomato
- 1 cup of oven-baked potato wedges
- 1 tsp Cajun spice
- 3 tbsp low-fat sour cream
- 1 tsp finely chopped fresh dill

Halve the burger bun and spread each half with Dijon mustard. Grill the bison burger patty and before stacking it on the bottom of the halved burger bun. Top the patty with a lettuce leaf, tomato slice, sliced pickle. In a bowl, mix together the sour cream and dill. Bake the potato wedges according to the pack, spice with Cajun spice and drizzle with the sour cream and fresh chive sauce.

Surf and Turf with a Baked Potato and Sour Cream - 500 Calories

- 1 prime cut steak - grilled and spiced to your liking
- 1 large baking potato, baked until soft
- 6 large grilled prawns
- 1 tsp garlic butter
- 1 tsp unsalted butter
- 1 tbsp sour cream
- 1 cup cooked green beans

Cook the steak and baking potato to your liking. Grill the prawns and heat the garlic butter when the prawns are nearly cooked. Cook the green beans to your liking and serve them onto a dinner plate. Add the steak, prawns, and baked potatoes. Pour the heated garlic butter over the prawns. Add unsalted butter, sour cream, salt, and pepper to the baked potato and serve while nice and hot.

Quick Black Bean Chili - 343 Calories

- ¼ cup of cooked brown rice
- ½ white onion chopped
- 2 large fresh tomatoes chopped
- 1 can black beans
- 2 tsp crushed garlic
- 1 tbsp of chili powder (strength to your taste)
- 2 tbsp of organic honey
- 2 tbsp jalapeno peppers
- 2 tbsp organic balsamic vinegar
- 2 tsp paprika
- 2 tbsp sour cream
- 4 tbsp of feta
- ½ thinly sliced avocado
- 8 sprigs of fresh mint
- ¼ cup of warm water

This recipe makes 4 servings.

Cook the rice when the chili has fifteen minutes of cooking time left. In a large pot bring the warm water to boil, add the onion, black beans, crushed garlic, chili powder, honey, balsamic vinegar, and paprika. Allow the chili to cook for 1 hour 30 minutes or until the beans are soft. Serve with a dollop of sour cream, crumbled feta, avocado, and some fresh mint.

Avocado, Bacon, Rocket, and Feta Tortilla Pizza - 342 Calories

- 1 whole wheat tortilla
- ¼ avocado thinly sliced
- ¼ cup crisped bacon pieces
- 4 tbsp rocket
- 2 tbsp feta
- 4 tbsp shredded mozzarella
- 2 tsp organic tomato paste
- low-sodium salt and black pepper to taste

Preheat the oven to 340°F. Spread the tortilla with tomato paste, top with mozzarella, avocado, bacon, rocket, and crumble the feta cheese over the top. Place it in the oven and cook until all the ingredients are cooked, and the tortilla is golden brown.

Spicy Mince Meat Pancakes - 370 Calories

- Make a pancake mixture (2 eggs, ¼ cup flour, ¼ cup reduced-fat milk)
- 1 cup mince
- 5 basil leaves
- 1 tsp dried oregano
- 1 tsp chili powder
- 1 tsp jalapeno peppers
- 1 tsp capers

- ¼ cup mixed salad leaves
- ¼ cucumber chopped
- 1 celery stalk chopped
- 1 tsp balsamic vinegar

Make two pancakes. Cook the mince with the herbs and spices. Dish the mince out evenly into the middle of each pancake. Add jalapeno peppers and capers to each pancake and serve. Toss the salad greens together (salad leaves, cucumber, and celery) then drizzle balsamic vinegar over them. Serve the pancakes with the green salad on the side.

Healthy Smoothies

These smoothies can be used to replace breakfast or lunch. They can also be used as a snack.

Smoothies are fun to make and you can experiment with different fruit, nut, and vegetable blends. Add different types of nut milk, nut creams, yogurt, and so on. They are always tastier when you add seeds.

Keep the ingredients healthy and within snack or meal calorie requirements. They are a great way to get all your nutrition requirements in for the day. They can also be taken as an on the go meal or snack.

Smoothies may only be drunk during normal eating periods or windows. As they are a snack that contains carbs they cannot be drunk during the fasting periods.

They are easy to make as you put all the ingredients into a blender, then blend until smooth and thick. Leftover smoothie mixture can be kept in an airtight container in the refrigerator for up to two days.

Smoothies with added protein powder are a great way to aid muscle recovery after a tough workout, long run, bike ride, etc. They can also give you that added boost of energy if you are feeling tired and run down.

Smoothie Ingredients

Smoothies can contain any fruit, berry, nut, seed, protein whey powder, yogurt, etc.

Fruit and berries can be either frozen or fresh. Avoid canned fruit or berries and check that the products do not have any added sugar, flavors, or colorants.

Here are a few examples of the most popular smoothie ingredients:

Berries

- Raspberries
- Blackberries
- Blueberries
- Strawberries

Fruit

- Banana (they are great for thickening and sweetening a smoothie)
- Avocado
- Pear
- Plum
- Peach
- Apple
- Pineapple
- Melon (yellow)
- Papaya
- Watermelon
- Grapes
- Pomegranate seeds

- Kiwi
- Mango
- Coconut

Nuts

- Cashews
- Macadamia
- Walnuts
- Almonds
- Pecan
- Pistachios
- Brazil nuts

Seeds

- Chia
- Sunflower
- Pinenut
- Pumpkin
- Sesame
- Fennel

Vegetables

- Kale
- Spinach
- Cabbage
- Broccoli
- Tomato
- Celery
- Carrot
- Raddish
- Horseradish
- Cucumber
- Spring onion

- Artichoke
- Garlic
- Rocket
- Capers

Herbs

- Mint
- Basil
- Oregano
- Parsley
- Ginger
- Rosemary
- Cardamom
- Mustard seeds
- Chives

Spices

- Turmeric
- Paprika
- Cayenne pepper
- Ground cinnamon
- Allspice
- Chili powder
- Chili seeds
- Ground ginger
- Garlic powder
- Cumin
- Dill
- Low sodium salt
- Black pepper
- White pepper
- Worcestershire sauce
- Soy sauce

- Hot sauce
- Tomato ketchup
- Mustard

Liquids

- Filtered water
- Ice cubes
- Almond milk
- Hemp milk
- Rice milk
- Oat milk
- Coconut milk
- Coconut cream
- Coconut water
- Low-fat milk
- Cream
- Fruit juice
- Vegetable juice

Other

- Vanilla essence
- Pure vanilla
- Organic Balsamic vinegar
- Curry powder
- Vegetable oil
- Protein whey powder (all flavors)
- Plain low-fat Greek yogurt
- Low-fat cream cheese
- Fat-free cottage cheese
- Flavored low-fat yogurt
- Sugar-free ice cream (all flavors)
- Raw organic cocoa powder
- Dark chocolate chips

- Dark chocolate blocks
- Organic honey
- Desiccated coconut
- Coconut flakes
- Fresh chilis

Smoothie Ideas

These are tasty smoothies that are full of good nutrition, taste great and 350 calories or under.

Avocado, Banana, Chocolate, and Ginger Smoothie - 312 Calories

- ½ banana
- ½ avocado
- 1 tbsp grated fresh ginger root
- 1 tsp sunflower seeds
- 1 tsp chia seeds
- 1 tsp vanilla extract
- ¼ cup unsweetened almond milk
- ¼ cup of filtered water

Peach, Blueberry Cheesecake Smoothie - 350 Calories

- ½ banana
- 1 peach
- ½ cup blueberries
- 1 tbsp sesame seeds
- 1 tbsp organic honey
- ½ cup low-fat milk
- ¼ cup of ice cubes
- ¼ cup sugar-free vanilla ice cream

The Green and Gold Smoothie - 124 Calories

- ½ banana
- ¼ cup kale
- ¼ cup baby spinach leaves
- ¼ cucumber
- ½ green bell pepper
- 1 tsp fresh dill
- 2 tsp turmeric
- ½ cup of filtered water
- ¼ cup unsweetened coconut water
- low-sodium salt and black pepper to taste

Berry, Nut, and Seed Coconut Cream Smoothie with a Zing - 319 Calories

- ¼ cup blackberries
- ¼ cup blueberries
- ¼ cup raspberries
- ¼ cup pomegranate seeds
- 1 tsp sunflower seeds
- 1 tsp fennel seeds
- 1 tsp sesame seeds
- 3 tsp raw cashew nuts
- 2 tsp pecan nuts
- 2 tbsp unsweetened shredded coconut
- 4 tbsp unsweetened coconut cream
- ¼ cup unsweetened almond milk
- ¼ cup of filtered water
- 3 tsp organic honey
- dash of cayenne pepper

Tomato Beet Vegetable Cocktail Smoothie - 154 Calories

- 1 carrot

- 2 celery stalks
- 2 medium tomatoes
- ¼ cup baby spinach leaves
- ½ green bell pepper
- ¼ cucumber
- ¼ cup grated fresh beets
- 3 tsp fresh basil
- ½ cup of filtered water
- ¼ cup fresh orange juice
- low-sodium salt and ground black pepper to taste

Tropical Coconut Cream and Ginger Smoothie - 350 Calories

- ½ cup of pineapple
- ½ banana
- ½ mango
- 1 kiwifruit
- ¼ papaya
- 1 tbsp unsweetened shredded coconut
- 1 tbsp grated ginger root
- 1 tsp ground cinnamon
- 2 tsp organic honey
- ¼ cup fresh orange juice
- ¼ cup fresh lime juice

Beverages During Fasting Periods

There are some beverages you can drink during fasting periods and some you must avoid. There are also substances that must not be added to any beverages during fast and substances that can be added.

Here are some ideas on what you should and should not be drinking during fasting periods.

Water

Water should be drunk continuously during the day even when you are not fasting.

Water is always best drunk as natural, filtered, or spring water that can be either carbonated or still.

You May Add

- Lemon
- Lime
- Cucumber slices
- The water can be carbonated

You May Not Add

- Artificial sweeteners
- Colorants
- Artificial flavors
- Fruit
- Berries

Tea

There are a few teas that should be avoided and those that can be consumed. It is best to drink the tea black with a bit of cold water if it needs to be cooled down.

You May Drink the Following Tea

- Oolong tea
- Black tea
- Normal tea
- Green tea
- Cinnamon tea
- Peppermint tea

- Spearmint tea

- Stevia
- Cinnamon
- Nutmeg
- Lemon juice

You May Not Add

- Artificial sweeteners
- Milk
- Cream
- Artificial flavors
- Fruit
- Herbs
- Spices

Coffee

Black coffee helps to keep you alert and awake. It also can aid in weight loss.

You May Add

- Stevia
- Cinnamon
- Nutmeg
- Lemon juice

You May Not Add

- Artificial sweeteners
- Milk
- Cream
- Artificial flavors
- Herbs

- Spices

Concerns During Fasting

One of the major causes of people giving up fasting is because they get headaches, feel nauseous, or cannot stave off hunger.

Here are a few tips to help get you through a few concerns.

Constipation

Constipation does happen during fasting, especially when you first start out.

Try these tips:

- Increase your fiber content during your eating windows.
- Drink carbonated water.
- Use fennel seeds with your smoothies or sprinkle them over your food.
- Drink hot coffee.
- Drink black or green tea.

Dizziness

You may feel a bit dizzy or like you have vertigo during the fasting periods. You may even feel light-headed every time you stand up or get a blood rush to the head. This is usually caused by dehydration.

Try these tips:

- Increase your fluid intake.
- Drink mint in your water during the eating windows.
- Take liver salts during the eating window.
- Cut down on coffee and tea intake for a while.

Fatigue or Lethargy

You will feel a bit fatigued or lethargic during fasting periods. You could also be lacking some vital nutrients. Increase your nutrient intake during non-fasting periods.

Try these tips:

- Increase your fluid intake.
- Eat high energy foods during your eating window and at least an hour before your fasting period is about to start.
- Splash cold water on your face.
- Do some light exercise.
- Take supplements during your eating window.

Headaches

Headaches are another common occurrence during fasting. Your body goes through a period of withdrawal and is not used to being starved of food.

Try these tips:

- Drink more water.
- Drink mineral water during your non-fasting periods.

Muscle Cramps or Spasms

Fasting also means cutting down salt and some minerals. This can cause muscle cramps and muscle spasms.

Try these tips:

- Take Epsom salts twice a week during your eating windows.
- Increase your magnesium intake during your eating windows.

Nausea

You may experience nausea if hunger sets in or you may experience migraine symptoms.

Try these tips:

- Drink peppermint tea.
- Drink liver salts during your eating window.

Hunger

The most common concern or complaint is feeling hungry. There is a lot you can do to stop you from feeling hungry and to relieve the hunger pangs.

Try these tips:

- Increase your fiber content during your eating windows.
- Eat more slow-release carbs at least an hour before the fasting period begins.
- Drink carbonated water.
- Drink green tea.
- Drink coffee.
- Add cinnamon to your coffee or tea.
- Distract yourself by keeping busy with a hobby.
- Get some light exercise in or go for a long walk.
- Meditate.
- Go visit a friend.

Sleeping Problems

If you are fasting during the night you would have probably started fasting around 7:30 pm. Move that up to at least 9 pm and have a light snack and cup of chamomile tea before bed.

Read a book and turn off all electronics that may be disturbing your sleeping pattern. Make sure your room is cool, even in winter your room needs to be cool in order to maintain a quality sleep pattern.

Keep a fresh bottle of water next to your bed in case you get thirsty during the night so you do not have to get up and go pour one.

Learn sleep meditation to relax your body and help you drift off to sleep.

Chapter 8:
Maintaining Your Weight

Intermittent fasting should become a way of life and once you have started it, you should try to do it at least twice a month or every other month. After all, you are going to want to maintain your weight once you have reached your goal.

After Diet Natural Appetite Control

Once you have reached your goal weight, you will need to keep a maintenance diet plan. Try to keep your calories under control; at first it may seem like hard work, but it eventually becomes second nature.

Fasting should be on your list of things to do every now and then, or at least once a month. At first, when you start fasting, it is going to be hard, but persevere, drink water as it will help to keep you energized as well as awake.

If you keep fasting, you will soon start to feel the benefits of intermittent fasting. Your body will feel lighter, you will begin to be able to identify the signs of actual hunger. Once your body becomes used to fasting, you will be able to navigate fasting times without too much hunger. Eat food that keeps you fuller for longer and keep well hydrated, you will start to have more energy and feel healthier.

A natural way to contain hunger is to drink water before meals as it will fill you up and you will not eat too much. Try to cut back on snacks and only eat when you feel real hunger pangs. Instead of eating unhealthy snacks or sweets rather eat a piece of fruit or a handful of nuts.

Eat good carbs and whole foods instead of processed or sugary foods. For more energy, eat foods such as a banana's, avocado's, or a whole-wheat sandwich. These foods will keep you fuller for that much longer. Don't forget to hydrate, as water does wonders for the body, the skin, and even your hair. Listen to your body. It will let you know what it needs and the more you fast, the more in tune you will become with it.

Lowered Levels of Inflammation in the Body

The body is not really designed to have three large meals a day and then snacks in between. If we have learned anything from history, it is that our ancestors would go out foraging for food. There were times when food was in abundance and then times when it was not. So, they would either feast or go hungry for days at a time occasionally.

As they did not have the fancy tools or cooling equipment as we are fortunate to have these days, they could not store their food either. We do not only need sleep to keep us alert and give us downtime, we need it so our body can perform vital housekeeping functions. These housekeeping functions are made more difficult when we abuse our systems with bad food or too much food.

There have been studies that showed intermittent fasting caused an anti-inflammatory response in the body after fasting for certain periods of time. These anti-inflammatory responses include the following (Papconstantinou, 2019):

- Increase cellular immune response.
- Improve gut microbiota composition.
- Reduce the risk of insulin resistance.

It also reduces the risk of diabetes, rheumatoid arthritis, and Alzheimer's as it keeps them at bay by producing a chemical compound called β-hydroxybutyrate. This chemical compound is used by the cells to produce energy when the body hits a low blood sugar. It also helps the brain function better as well as the body's nervous system. Mostly it seems to keep the immune system in check, so it does not cause diseases as previously mentioned.

Inflammation is measured by cytokines, C-reactive protein markers which intermittent fasting helps to reduce.

Decreased Insulin Levels and Insulin Resistance

Studies have shown that fasting can significantly reduce body weight by up to 8% which is a start to getting insulin levels under control. The same studies showed that people who did alternate day fasting reduced their insulin levels by up to 52% and improved their insulin resistance by up to 53% (Arguin, Dionne, Sénéchal, Bouchard, Carpentier, Ardilouze, et al., 2012).

Although studies still continue and more research is needed before fasting will be clinically recommended, people who have followed an intermittent fasting diet have shown great results for a reduction in insulin levels and insulin resistance.

Clean Food for a Clean Mindset

Clean eating is a concept whereby a person makes themselves aware of where the food came from and how it got to their plate. In other words, eating foods that are not processed, and contain no GMOs or pesticides. Food not only has to be cooked in cleaner, more natural ways, but it has to have been handled that way before it was bought too.

Making the more natural and healthy choice when choosing your foods means cutting out boxed, packaged, processed, bagged, or artificially colored and flavored foods. Instead of going for the can of fruit choose the organic fresh fruit. But people who have followed an intermittent fasting diet have shown great results for reduction in insulin levels and insulin resistance.

These foods are called whole foods and include fresh foods, whole grains, unrefined sugars, less dairy, and lower salt. All of which is a lot healthier, reduces the risk of disease, and improves a person's overall health. After a person becomes familiar with and used to fasting, they will want to make healthier choices as they start to feel cleaner on the inside.

At first, you may think it is quite the mission to make these choices but if you persevere and take the extra minute to read the back of a can or package you will notice all the added ingredients. Most of which you probably cannot even pronounce, and they are not natural. You are making the effort to become healthier, lose weight, and feel better so go the extra mile and make those better food choices.

Once you have tasted the difference in whole foods over-processed, refined, and artificially grown, flavored, or colored you will naturally avoid them. Eating clean reprograms both your mind and body to want cleaner foods.

Chapter 9:
Intermittent Fasting Foods

It is very, very important to hydrate while intermittent fasting as the body will process the sugar that is stored in the liver (glycogen) to burn as an energy source. When it burns glycogen, the body also loses a large volume of fluid which needs to be replenished.

Water is the best hydration for the body, and a person should drink at least the recommended daily dose of it, more if you are doing a lot of exercise.

Some of the foods and beverages to eat or drink when fasting should include:

- Unsweetened tea and coffee must be drunk without any flavoring or powdered milk substitutes.
- Water is the best beverage to drink as long as it is plain water with no flavoring. You can infuse the water with mint but cannot add anything to sweeten it.
- You will need carbohydrates to sustain you through the fasting periods so during the eating window try to eat whole grains.
- Potatoes constitute another significant source of food for the body and most white potatoes are easily digested by the body. They also promote good gut bacteria to help your digestion.
- Chickpeas are a very versatile food and can be eaten as a roasted snack or as hummus.
- Fruit, and vegetables (or a mixture of both) smoothies made with nut milk fill the body with needed nutrients and can also take away sweet cravings. They are filling

and as long as you stick to healthy choices you can experiment with the flavors.

- Berries are a great snack and are so healthy, they are packed full of goodness. Try blueberries, raspberries, and blackberries. They are also filled with antioxidants and are another way of quelling sweet cravings.
- Nuts, eaten in moderation, are a great snack; they also complement many dishes. They aid the body in eliminating fat; they can also reduce the risk of type 2 diabetes and may increase longevity.
- Supplements are something to consider as you may not be consuming enough nutrients.
- Dairy products that are fortified with vitamin D as this is the one vitamin that most people tend to lack. You can get vitamin D by exposing your skin to at least 15 minutes in the sun a day. But there are places in the world where that is just not possible for long periods of the year. So look for healthy products that possess an adequate amount of vitamin D, which a lot of fortified milk products have.

Intermittent Fasting Foods to Control Blood Sugar Levels

To control insulin levels during intermittent fasting, a person should include the following foods into their daily diet and eating windows:

- Fatty fish such as herring, salmon, sardines, mackerel, and anchovies contain a good quantity of Omega 3 fats. Fatty fish may lower a person's risk of heart disease as well as being good for blood sugar levels. It is also good for brain power as well as cuts down inflammation markers in the body.

- Eggs, not only help to reduce insulin levels but they are also one of the best foods to eat to keep a person fuller for longer. They are also good for reducing the risk of heart disease; it feeds the muscles, improves insulin resistance, and decreases inflammation markers.
- Greek yogurt is another food that helps to reduce blood sugar levels. It is also a very versatile food that can be used to replace mayonnaise. It can be used to thicken smoothies, replace ice cream, eaten as a dish on its own, or enjoyed as a dessert topped with berries.
- Strawberries are at the top of the list when it comes to nutritious fruits. They are very high in antioxidants, especially the one that gives them their color called anthocyanin. Anthocyanin may reduce the risk of heart disease, reduce cholesterol, and can lower blood sugar after a meal.
- Nuts contain fiber. They also have low digestible carbs which make them a great low-carb option. There are some nuts though that are a bit more carbs than others. But a person should include cashews, Brazil nuts, hazelnuts, almonds, pistachio, walnuts, and pecans.
- Turmeric is something that a person should try to incorporate into their meal even if they do not need to control blood sugar. It has cancer-fighting properties as well as reduces the risk of heart disease besides being a natural component for controlling insulin levels.
- Seeds such as flax seeds have great fiber in them to help reduce insulin levels. Chia seeds are another great seed source filled with fiber and compounds that not only reduce insulin but also the risk of heart disease and cancer.
- Leafy green vegetables like spinach, lettuce, and kale help to control insulin levels while also reducing the

risk of heart disease. They are also packed with vitamins and nutrients that the body needs, especially during fasting.

- Garlic is not just to add flavor to a meal it has many great health properties to it as well. These include helping to control insulin levels, fighting cancer, and reducing the risk of heart disease.
- Cinnamon should somehow be inserted into a person's daily diet as it has so much to offer. One benefit, in particular, is that it helps to control insulin levels after meals.
- Squash is a food that does not get all the mention it should. All kinds of squash such as butternut, pumpkin, zucchini, and various summer squashes to help not only control insulin levels but obesity too.
- Broccoli is another food that a lot of people really do not like. They prefer to go for cauliflower. While cauliflower has its benefits, broccoli is an easily digestible carb that contains vitamins C along with other much-needed nutrients and vitamins.

Detox Food for Energy and Vitality

Some foods can help in detoxing the system. Then there are those foods a person should avoid if trying to detox.

Foods to avoid include:

- Dairy products are acidic which can slow down the detoxification process as these products can lead to the cells not functioning as they should.
- Alcohol should be avoided at all costs as it is toxic and affects the liver. Alcohol reduces levels of magnesium and zinc which are products needed for detoxification.
- Meat does not get digested very fast and promotes the breeding of bacteria in the gut. This bacteria is not the

good kind either. Meat tends to clog up the system as it is hard for the body to digest so it takes longer, thus slowing down the digestion.

- Caffeine is also harmful as it has been known to increase toxicity in the body.
- Salt is also not too good for the body and can raise a person's blood pressure. High blood pressure causes a lot of damage and increases the risk of a stroke. It is not good for detoxing either as it slows down normal cell function.
- Sugar should be avoided, especially processed sugar. Even brown sugar that is not organic has been processed. It also conflicts with the good bacteria in a person's gut which can be detrimental for detoxing. While sugar may give a person an instant rush of energy, it burns off really quickly which could leave you feeling drained afterward. It is also quite addictive as your body comes to crave the sugar rush.
- Avoid packaged foods or foods with artificial colors or flavors. Foods that contain a lot of salt or saturated fats must also be avoided.

Food to eat to encourage detox and boost your energy levels includes:

- Vegetables; if you can try to find organic vegetables and choose fresh rather than frozen.
- Berries are high in antioxidants. Fresh berries are always the better choice. Although frozen berries are just as good if sugar-free and with little to no preservatives.
- Whole grains are high in fiber which promotes gut health to aid digestion and keeps you feeling full.
- Most fruit is a great source of natural sugar. They not only aid in detoxing but also help to stave off sweet

cravings. They are also full of vital vitamins and nutrients.

- Nuts and seeds are a great source of protein help to improve detoxing. They also contain many healthy nutrients. They also contain fat-soluble vitamins vital for feeding the brain.

Anti-Aging Foods

One of the first places to show an indication of a problem within the human body is the skin. It is after all the largest organ of the body. A person can use all the topical lotions as well as potions but there is only so much they can do. The skin needs to heal and be rejuvenated from within the body through feeding it correctly.

One of the best ways to reduce fine lines, smooth out wrinkles, or eliminate those dark spots or lines is through eating correctly. A bright healthy glowing skin comes from within not from some potion or magical base cover you have applied to it.

To help encourage healthy skin and slow down the signs of aging your diet should include the following foods:

- Blueberries are supercharged foods that contain a good number of vitamins A and C. They also contain anthocyanin which is an antioxidant with age-defying properties. Blueberries are also a great way to sweeten plain yogurt or smoothies.
- Avocado contains some nutrients that have been known to slow down the effects of aging. These nutrients are potassium, vitamin K, vitamin C, Vitamin A, and B vitamins. They also contain helpful carotenoids that aid in stopping the harmful effects of the sun which in turn may help fight against skin cancer.

- Papaya is a superfood that contains a high content of minerals, vitamins, and antioxidants to improve the skin's appearance. Papaya may just be the superfood required to smooth out those fine lines or wrinkles and improve the skin's elasticity. It is also a rich source of vitamins E, vitamin K, vitamin A, vitamin C, potassium, calcium, magnesium, and B vitamins. It is one of the foods you should be trying to eat at least once or twice a week.
- Nuts and seeds make the list again as some nuts, like walnuts, contain Omega-3 fatty acids. Omega-3 has been known to help protect the skin against the harmful rays of the sun, create a natural glow, and help to strengthen the skin membranes.
- Pomegranate is another superfood that most people are unaware of but has been used in alternative medicines for centuries. They contain punicalagin which helps in the slowing down of the skin aging process as it protects collagen.
- Red bell peppers contain lots of vitamin C. Vitamin C is essential for the production of collagen. They also contain carotenoids which are well-known antioxidants.
- Leafy green vegetables, broccoli, and sweet potatoes are also vegetables that help to maintain the skin as they contain lots of vitamins and nutrients. These vitamins and nutrients are particularly helpful in protecting the skin from the harmful damage of the sun.

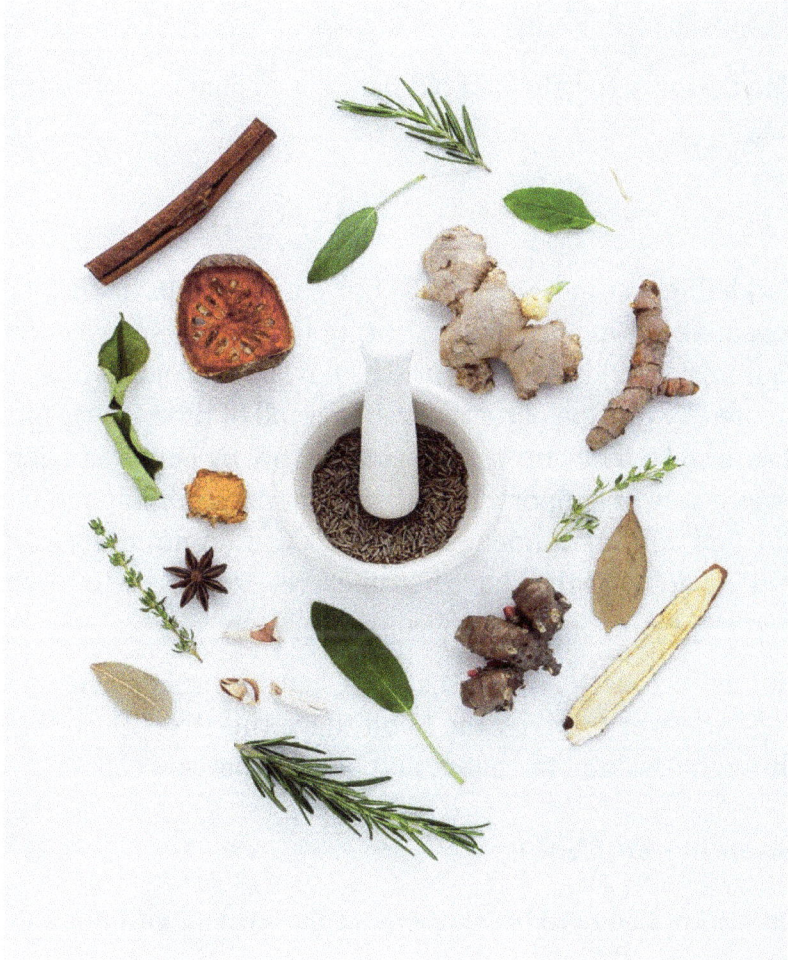

Chapter 10:
Changing Your Habits and Your Mindset to Change Your Body

The best way to get rid of old habits is to change your mindset.

Take Control of Your Habits

Bad habits get ingrained into your subconscious as they are repeated day in and day out. Biting your nails, sucking your thumb, eating three large meals a day, and so on. Habits are created by routine patterns over a period of time. These habits are started by our parents growing up, by nerves, anxiety, or as a way of support. Breaking them does not happen in a day and will take time. Some habits you do not even know you are doing as they have become a reflex. This includes the way you eat, cook, and even shop.

Habits, no matter what they are, can be broken. You just need to want to break the habit, have the strength to push through breaking the habit, and believe that you can.

Breaking Bad Habits

Instead of trying to break them, replace them with healthier ones.

Here are some tips on how to take control of your habits in order to change them.

The Triggers

Become aware of your triggers. Once you are aware of why you do what you do, you can find a way around them. Habits are a person's little comfort devices and as such are really easy to fall back into. In order to change them, we need to develop new comforts and at midlife, it becomes quite a challenge to do.

One way to retrain the response to a trigger would be to have a countermeasure in place. For example, if you find yourself reaching for dessert after supper, stop and ask yourself why you are having the dessert. Are you still hungry? If so, go get something with less sugar and calories in, or reach for fruit instead.

If you are really wanting something sweet, have a glass of infused water and think about what healthy snacks you could eat instead. Grapes are a healthier alternative to sweets, chocolates, or carbonated drinks.

Don't think, "I must eat something healthy." Rather think, "I would much prefer something healthy to eat."

When you go shopping, don't think, "I must prefer to take this product." Reach for the healthier alternative and think "Ah! This is my new favorite brand."

Dealing with Triggers

Most people are aware of their triggers on some level. The best solution would be to avoid situations that trigger bad habits. The thing is, in real life you are always going to come across a trigger or two somewhere. It is like trying to avoid a person you do not like, unless you are going to change continents, even then that is no guarantee.

If you cannot avoid them, learn how to deal with them. As per the section above, have a coping mechanism you can fall back on other than the bad habit. If you find you are unable to resist hotdogs, when you pass a hotdog vendor carry a nutritious snack with you. A few squares of dark chocolate could do the trick or a handful of berries or nuts. Take it out and eat it as you pass by or dial a friend to occupy your mind while you walk past.

Find a mantra that best suits you and talk yourself through it when you find yourself in a situation that triggers a habit. You are trying to combat the signs of aging, not just on the outside but on the inside. To do that you have to break the bad eating habits and that includes the way you cook, the groceries you buy, and eating out habits. Most decent restaurants and even fast-food places are trying to offer healthy menu choices. Think of trying something new on the menu for a new and improved you!

Switching the Bad for the Good

In theory, it sounds quite easy to do but in reality, it is really hard. You have spent most of your life eating the way you do, shopping the way you do, and so on. By now your life works on autopilot as you go through your habitual daily routine. Now you are trying to slowly change your entire lifestyle and undo all those years of mental wiring.

It is going to take strength, commitment, and perseverance. But the end results of intermittent fasting and opting for a healthier lifestyle really do justify the means. One of the best ways to start is to think of it as switching out this product for a new product. Kind of like switching out your laundry detergents to try a new brand. Don't think of it as breaking bad habits or a diet. Rather think of your new lifestyle as trying something new.

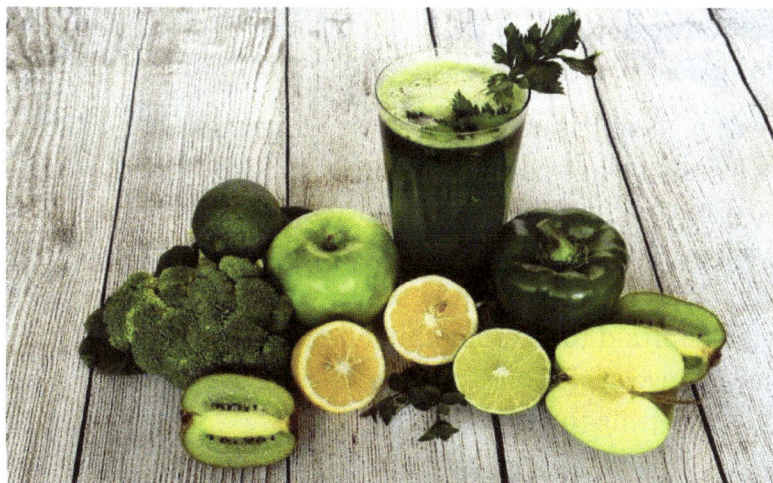

Change Your Mindset

You have had a certain mindset for years and now you are changing it. Retraining your brain, setting new routines, and developing new comfort zones. The human psyche is complex, and humans really are their own worst enemies. Believe it or not, you are going to come up against resistance to all your changes. Even the smallest of changes may have some form of resistance. The hardest part is it is not resistance from a moody teenager or partner. The resistance to change will come from within you!

You can start to change your mindset by trying some of the following methods:

Have a Clear Vision

One thing on your side, when you reach midlife, is that your taste changes. Usually, at midlife, a person starts to find that foods that once agreed with them no longer do. While other foods may become more appealing, your tastes can actually change and food may not taste the same. Now is the best time to embrace new eating habits. You have the perfect excuse to use against your inner rebel.

If eating meat has started to cause indigestion, try substituting it with a plant-based alternative. Chickpeas make a great, tasty, meat alternative. If you love bacon, you don't have to give it up entirely; once again try a plant alternative, like eggplant. Find the foods that best suit you and your new tastes, don't be afraid to try something new. This is a new phase of your life cycle. Not only are you turning over a new leaf, but you are getting to know this new you.

Parents will have gone through the different phases in their kid's life and as they grew you had to grow with them. You adapted and evolved around the different stages. This is a lot like that, only now you have reached a new phase of your life. To enjoy your golden years in optimum health, change is necessary. Even those that have led a relatively healthy lifestyle, trained every day, and conquered mountains, will have to adapt at this point in their life.

Your body is changing from the inside, and what worked for you before menopause will most likely no longer work for you now. You can't let it defeat you or get you down, you need to embrace it and set your vision as to where you go from here. Make a list of the most significant changes you feel you need to address. Include what you would like to change and note any health issues that you feel you need to address.

Midlife Vision Board

Vision boards are a lot of fun and are really trending these days. They give you something to aspire to and as you notice changes during your lifestyle change it serves as a great visualization tool. There is nothing more motivating than actually seeing the changes and how much you have transformed from point A to where you currently are.

Chart Your Progress

Set a date for once a week, bi-weekly, or monthly where you take note of your changes. Weigh yourself, measure yourself, take note of much further you can walk now, and so on. Document how you feel. Are you sleeping better? Do you feel like you have more energy now?

List all the changes you made for the time period, how you adapted to them, and any new changes or modifications you think you need.

Make sure to write down the times you slipped up, anything you had a hard time with and the things that just did not meet your needs. It may seem like hard work, but you will be amazed how encouraging it is when you lay it all out. It also gives you a baseline from which to work from and a way to make adjustments.

Set Obtainable Goals

One of the worst things you can do is set your targets or goals too high. Keep a clear vision in mind of what your overall target is. Then set weekly or rather monthly targets to strive for.

Make weekly goals about small adjustments to your lifestyle, like changing dairy products for nut milk. Make your monthly targets about losing weight or rather centimeters and your fitness levels.

Breaking down your lifestyle goals into smaller obtainable and doable chunks makes achieving your overall goal more realistic. Having small goals is similar to breaking down a project into milestones. You know where the project is going and how it should end up and the steps to take to get there.

Having smaller goals helps keep up your morale because there is nothing like achieving that first milestone. That is when you know you are on the right path, and it makes you want to get to the next milestone.

It also keeps you in a positive can-do mindset as once you have reached the next few, you are well on your way to the final goal post.

A New Daily Routine

When you change your eating habits, it affects your daily routine, especially when intermittent fasting. You have to schedule your meals around your fasting days as well as your social calendar. If you are unsure if you will be able to resist temptation, it is best to schedule family outings, lunches, and get-togethers on non-fasting days. There are, obviously, going to be times when you cannot do this. Instead, try to be flexible regarding your scheduled fasting days instead.

Your Daily To-Do List

You need to organize your schedule in order to start a new routine. The first thing you should do is create your daily task list. This is everything you do throughout the day and which days you do what tasks on.

While fasting should not interfere with your daily routine, it could possibly interfere with your social one. In order to benefit from intermittent fasting, you need to make it fit into your life. To choose or modify a plan to best suit your needs, you need to establish what your current routine is so you can adapt it to fit your new lifestyle.

While jotting down what all you do during the day each day, here are some questions to keep in mind:

- How does the morning start? Write down the general time you get up. Any pre-breakfast tasks?

- Do you make breakfast every morning?
- Do you have kids you need to get off to school, college, or work?
- Do you have a partner that needs to get off to work?
- If you are working, what is your morning routine to get ready?
- Do you have any work function commitments in the next one to three months?
- Do you have any social or family functions/gatherings/commitments within the next three months?
- When are grocery days?
- When are laundry days?
- What housework do you do and when?
- Do you exercise? If so, how frequently?
- What hobbies do you have?
- Do you have a club membership and are there any club engagements coming up?
- List any events you may have coming up, holidays, sports tournaments, sport commitments, and so on.

Include everything that you may think is relevant to your schedule that you know you do like clockwork. Events such as weddings, engagement parties, birthday functions, work functions all need to be jotted down. As do any social engagements, book clubs, girls' nights out, etc. They all play a crucial part in having a well-adjusted fasting schedule that works well with and for you.

Create a New Schedule

Choose the type of fasting plan you think you may be able to start with and stick to. Before you commit to time windows for fasting and eating, assess your current schedule. You will need to adjust your schedule and maybe even modify your fasting plan to find a compromise for your schedule.

Before you start making up your schedule, it is time to take stock of you. Note the times of day you feel you have the highest energy levels. This is the time of day to do the heavy lifting, like exercises and training your mind to break old habits to make room for new ones. Use your afternoons to set up menus for the next day, make appointments, go watch the kid's sports games or meet up with friends for tea.

Do things that do not require a lot of energy, but that still keep you active and your mind working.

You should include a number of things on your schedule like:

- The time you need to wake up each morning so you can set your alarm.
- Any appointments you, your partner, or kids may have each day.
- Shopping for groceries, or any household, school, or office supplies you may need.
- Family commitments for the day or evening.
- Upcoming events you need to get yourself and your family ready for.
- New foods you would like to try each day.
- Any changes you would like to make on certain days that will ease you into your new healthy lifestyle.
- Exercise for the day.
- Set a time window for bedtimes. This may seem a bit infantile, but you need to start getting a decent sleep pattern going. If you make a concerted effort to get to bed at a regular time each night, your body will soon adapt to this routine. You will find yourself starting to feel tired by a certain point of the evening.

Wake Up with a Smile

The most popular time of day for high-energy levels is when you first wake up. This is the time your body should be well-rested and restored. This is the time of day you should be the most active and enjoy your energy. Make the most of the time to go for a walk, get the major part of your tasks done before your energy levels start to get depleted.

Train yourself to wake up with the correct attitude. Wake up with the first ring of your alarm — do not hit that snooze button. Have a big stretch to get the blood flowing through your system and get up, don't be tempted to laze in your bed. Your attitude upon waking will set the tone for the entire day.

Not everyone is a morning person but resetting the alarm is resetting your brain into old habits. It is as if you are putting off waking up for the day and you need to change that to be more positive. Even if you feel a bit blah at first, take a deep breath, stretch and hop out of bed. Smile if only to yourself in the mirror as a smile is infectious and makes everyone feel better.

A refreshing shower is a good way to get yourself going in the morning and it makes you feel alive. It is a symbolic way to wash away the sleepiness from the night before and step out of the shower cleansed for the new day. Splashing cold water on your face and neck will stimulate the Vagus nerve and kick start your morning as well.

Be Active Throughout the Day

You may not feel like it as your energy levels start to get depleted but don't slow down altogether. Don't take an afternoon nap either, that may just make you feel even more lethargic and can cause problems by disturbing your nightly sleep patterns.

If you work in an office environment, take a break every thirty minutes where you actually get up and go get a glass of water. Stand up and stretch, roll your neck, and stretch out your feet. Get your blood pumping through your veins and take some deep breaths.

If you are at home, go for a walk around the garden and check out your plants. Or go for a walk in the park, feed the ducks and take in some fresh air. Do a puzzle or play Candy Crush for fifteen minutes to get your brain stimulated as well.

As long as you are keeping your mind ticking and pushing through the feeling of lethargy that may creep up on you in the afternoons. If you can push through it, you will eventually find you will start to have a little more afternoon energy each afternoon.

Going for a swim and getting some gentle exercise even when you feel like your body just wants to collapse is a good way to get the adrenaline flowing through your system. If you must close your eyes, have a small five- to eight-minute power nap. You will be surprised how refreshed you can feel when you close your eyes and let yourself relax for shorter periods of time.

The Evenings

It is important to make evenings the time of day when you put away all the stress and anxieties of the day. When you walk through the front door or notice the clock turn six, it is time to shut out the day. Concentrate on what you have to do in the evening, like getting supper going, change into comfortable clothes, and maybe get ready for the next day.

Once you have had your evening meal, which you should try to eat by 7:30 pm each day, plan your next day. Decide on your meals, get your clothes ready, take a shower to wash off the day then take time to relax. Watch a bit of TV or read a good book or just have a chat with your partner and kids.

Make evenings about family, you, and getting organized for tomorrow. Leave the worrying about the next day for the next day. Evenings are the time you need to learn to unwind to allow for good quality sleep. When you do not get enough sleep, it makes it difficult to successfully fast, or get through your next day.

Give Yourself Room to Be Flexible

Having a set routine is a good thing but that does not mean you have to be completely rigid with it. Remember to give yourself a little bit of room for error. Your body needs to adjust to its new lifestyle so give yourself some time. Keep an open mind and learn how to quickly adjust and adapt to any situations that may arise.

You can have your routines and comfort zones but don't forget to be a little spontaneous too. Life is not all boring mundane routines it is also about living and during your golden years is the time to enjoy life.

Let go once in a while, listen to your body and follow its lead.

Setting up new routines is going to take getting used to. Some things may not work at first so adjust them until they do work for you and you find them easy to follow. Changing your mindset is not about creating problems or making life more difficult for you. It is about finding a new balance that works just as smoothly as the old one did. Only the new one is setting you up for a new healthier you with clean eating habits.

Deep down we all wish we could have a perfect life that ran smoothly like clockwork. But the reality is that life can be messy and no matter how perfectly we plan it, it does not always go according to plan. Keep your goals and schedules real, achievable and flexible. You cannot plan for everything, but there are certain things that you can plan for. The things that you can't, you will have to deal with as they happen. As you adjust to a healthier lifestyle, you will find the unexpected a lot easier to deal with without the foggy brain or run-down feeling.

Those things you can plan for, you don't need to set them in stone, just have a good idea of how you are going to deal with them.

It Is All Up to You

Reading self-help books, laying out the groundwork, and setting goals is the easy part. The hard part is putting it all into practice and that is all up to you. Now that you have chosen your fasting plan, decided upon a diet, and set your new routine, it is time to take the next step.

It is time to get real and set a realistic start date. Go to bed the night before and think about sleep as your cocoon. The next morning you are going to wake up taking on the first day of your new lifestyle. The new you is about to start blossoming and become healthier, stronger, and more confident.

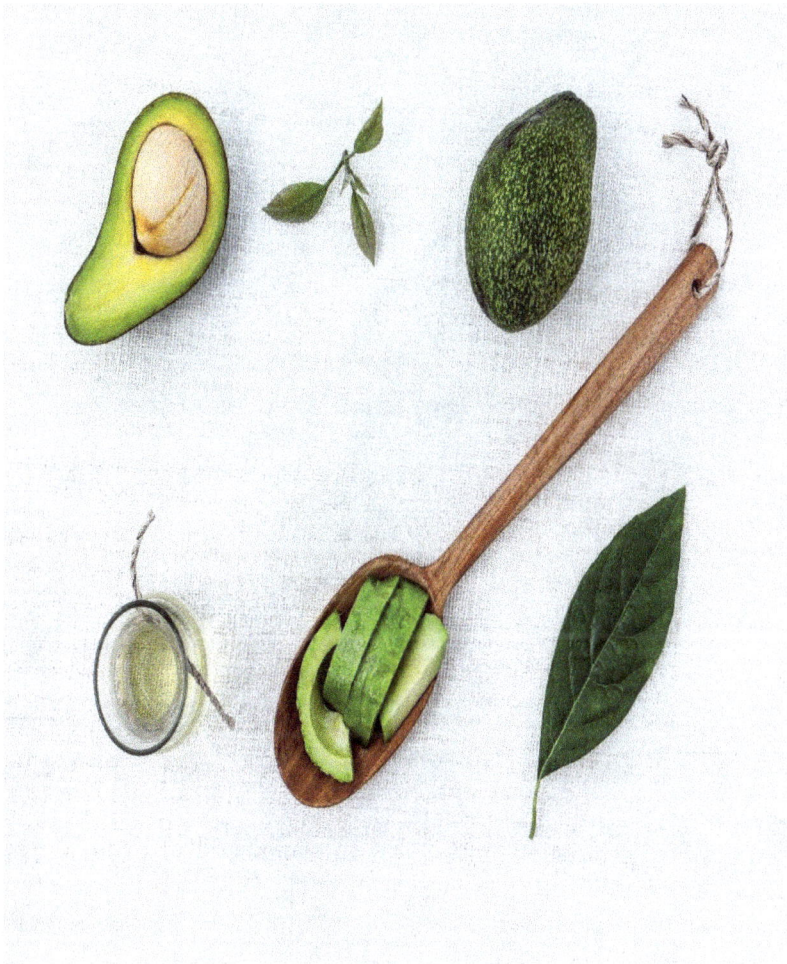

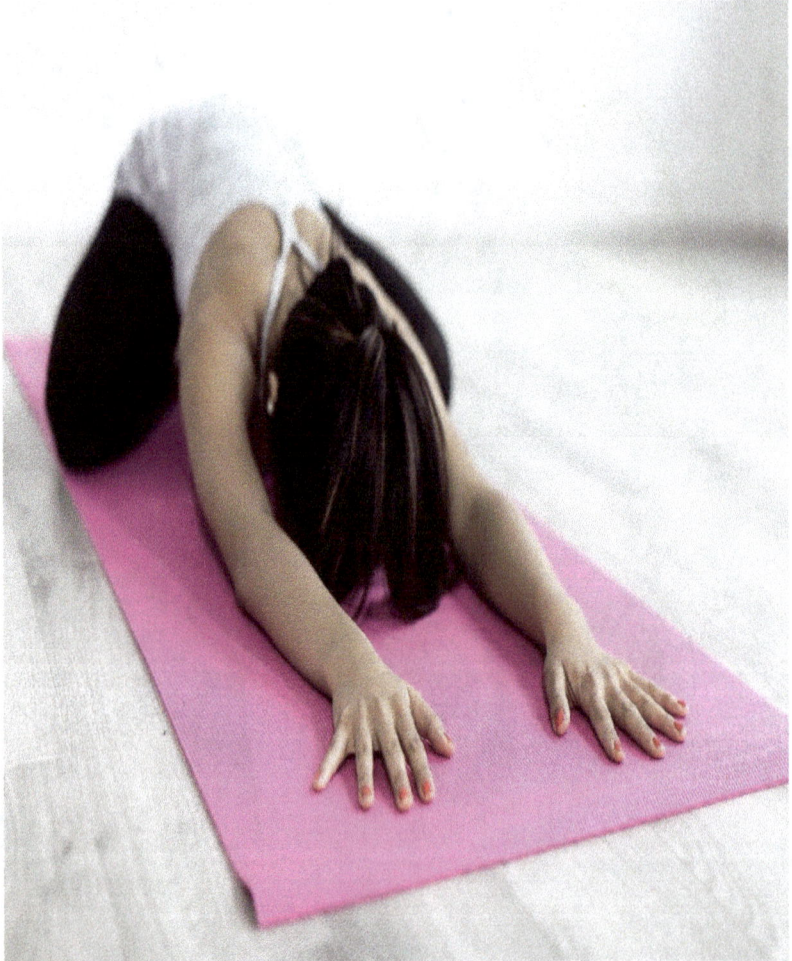

Chapter 11:
Reaching Your Goals

It takes a lot of hard work and staying power. Once you have reached your goal weight, dropped a dress size or two there is no greater feeling.

You Made It!

When you have come so far, it is cause for celebration and everyone deserves to have a bit of fun, let their hair down and reward themselves. As long as you do not fall back into old habits and keep a maintenance plan that maintains your weight as well as your health.

You Are What You Eat

When you have reached your goal weight, you will feel healthier, have more energy, and look great. You may even have a glow about you as your system is cleansed and has probably been kick-started to work at its optimum level. Be mindful of what you eat and keep up the good habits of grabbing the healthier options of your favorite foods.

New Lifestyle, New You

A healthier lifestyle is the best change you can make. Your healthier choices and intermittent fasting lifestyle will become the new you. You may not be the same girl you once were, but now you are an incredible woman. You are stronger, more confident and a whole lot healthier.

Enjoy Your Success

When you feel good you will look good and will be able to wear your new-found confidence with pride. And you earned it so enjoy your midlife years, they are nothing to be ashamed of but rather are to be enjoyed. You have passed all the awkward years, you are over all of your insecurities, and now you get to be you. A new, gorgeous, healthier you that glows from the inside out.

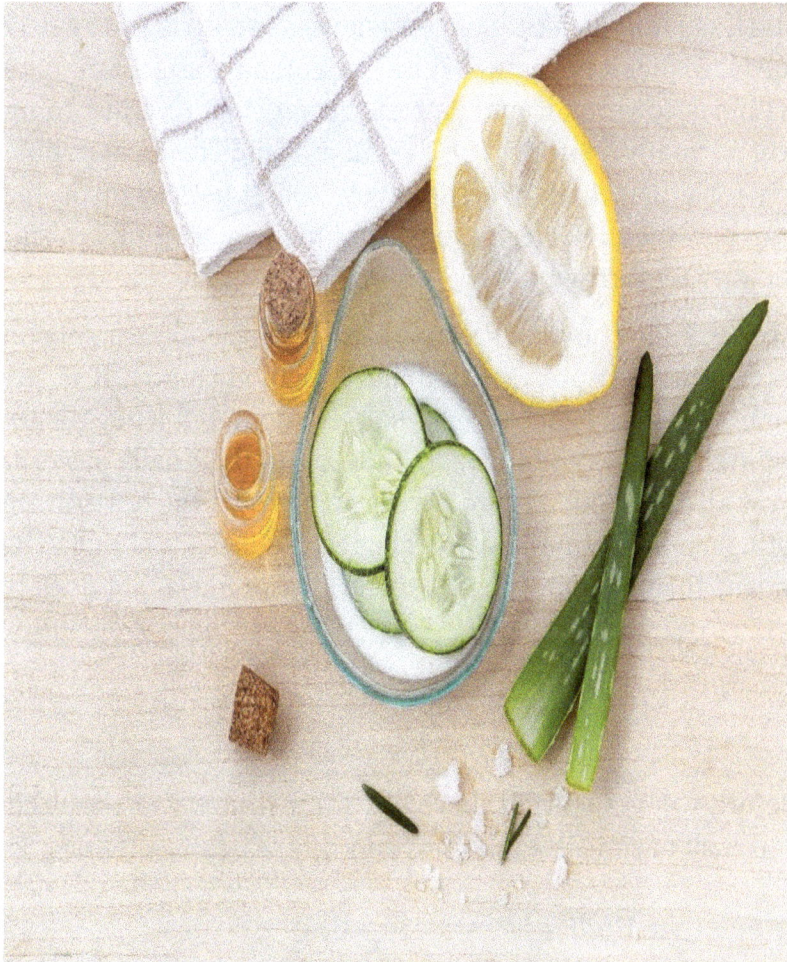

Chapter 12:
Getting Started

Starting a diet is a challenge because as soon as you register the word diet it becomes a mission. You have an instant mental block towards it and you may even start to crave things you normally do not eat on a regular basis. The most popular day for a diet to start is tomorrow. Don't get caught in that trap and eat all you can today thinking you are going to start the diet tomorrow.

Even thinking about a lifestyle change can send your subconscious into self-preservation and rebellious mode. It is easy for others to say get over yourself and do it, but a person gets set in their ways and for years they follow their daily patterns. Now all of a sudden there are big changes on the horizon and let's face it no one likes to change. Especially change that means turning your lifestyle upside down like a diet does.

Getting Ready to Embrace Your New Lifestyle

Before you get started there are a few things you should do and may need to get ready.

Speak to a Medical Professional

This is very important if you are on any kind of medication. If you have a pre-existing condition or are ill in any way, you should not try fasting without the guidance of a medical professional.

It is a good idea to get a medical checkup before you start a diet. Even young adults should always start a diet getting the all-clear from a doctor.

Choose a Fasting Plan

If you are starting out with intermittent fasting, choose a plan that is not too limiting. For instance, the 5:2 plan with a 12-hour fasting period and a 12-hour eating window to begin with. You could try the 16-hour fasting period and 8-hour eating window if you think you will cope.

If you find the plan is too much for you, switch it for another one or modify the one you are on. Build yourself up to a longer fasting period. As long as you are moving forward and not going backward with your fasting plan.

Set achievable goals and make sure you give yourself some wiggle room as well as being prepared for the times you may slip.

Make a calendar and place it where you can see it, mark your fasting and non-fasting days as well as time windows on it.

Keep an intermittent fasting diary, log how you felt during fasting, any changes you have found within yourself, improvements, days you may have fallen off the fasting wagon. It is important to document the process as it demonstrates your commitment and it will inspire you.

Be kind to yourself, you are going to have unpleasant days and good days. It is important to remember you are doing this for you. Don't feel guilty for one guilty pleasure now and then, just ensure they become less and less frequent..

Fasting Diet Plan

The best diet during the fasting period is to only drink un-sweetened, carb-free drinks like water, tea, and coffee. But there is nothing wrong with starting out with a 500 calorie allowance during the fasting period. Most people find it easier to fast through the night into the late morning.

Non-Fasting Day Eating Plan

Although there is no recommended diet for intermittent fasting, it is advisable to follow a healthy clean eating plan. Cut down on daily calorie intake, drink more water and choose fruit or nuts instead of sugary or processed foods. Make small changes and start switching out the unhealthy for more natural healthier products. Don't overthink the process and slowly you will rewire your brain to automatically reach for those foods.

Some good eating plans are a low-carb diet, calorie cycling plans like Weight Watchers, and becoming more aware of what you are eating. Make a point of thinking that you are what you eat, and you want to be healthy.

Breakfast

It has been drilled into a person since youth that breakfast is the most important meal of the day. But that does not mean you can't eat it at say 11 am; you are still eating breakfast.

It is believed that breakfast kick starts a person's metabolism to aid in the burning of calories throughout the day. There are other ways to kick start your metabolism like including a dash of cayenne pepper to your morning coffee. Cayenne pepper helps the body to burn calories for up to three hours after consuming it. First, check with your doctor before using

it as it can interfere with some medical conditions and med-
ications.

In general, it is not going to harm you to skip breakfast a few
times a week during a fasting period. Our ancestors did not
get up every morning to a bowl of porridge or a three-egg
omelet. Your body will soon adjust to its new routine, and
you will start missing your morning meal less.

Charged with Optimism

"Whatever the mind can conceive and believe, the mind can
achieve" — (Hill, 1937).

Start your new intermittent fasting lifestyle off on an optimistic note. Go into the diet fully charged and ready to go.
Psych yourself up mentally and enthusiastically think of this
change as going on a holiday from the old you and embrace
this journey you have embarked upon.

If you believe you can do it, you will do it. Just keep pushing
through the tough days, enjoy the good days, and forgive the
slip-ups. Eventually, you will be having more good days than
bad until you have completely turned your lifestyle around
and are reaping the benefits of it.

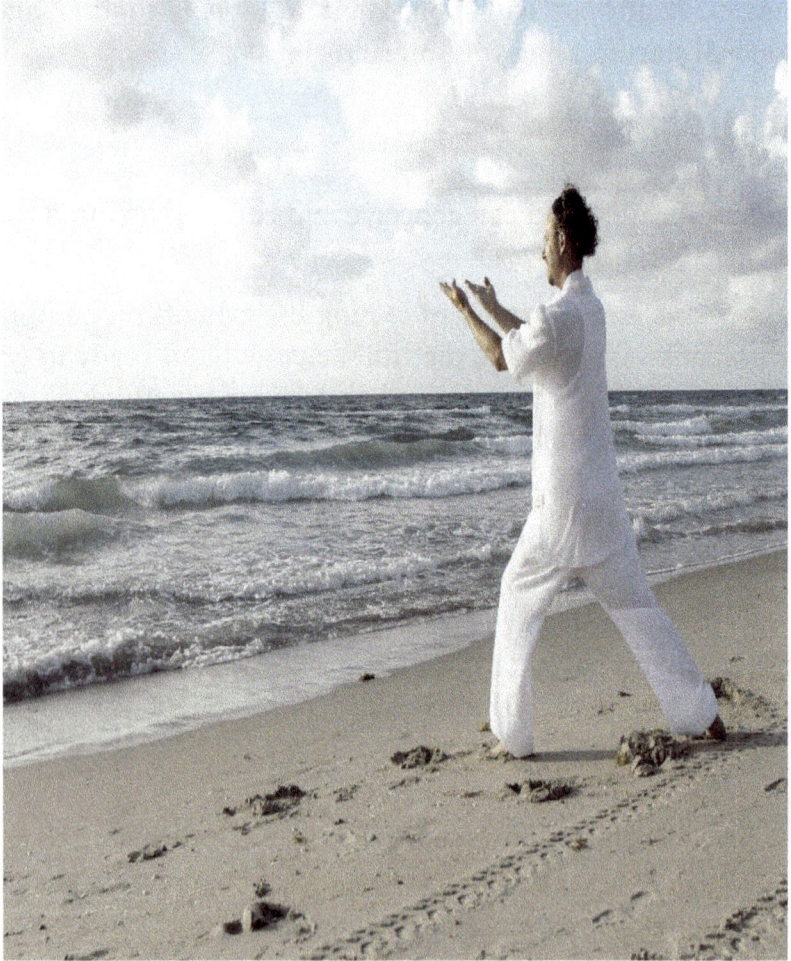

Conclusion

Intermittent fasting can be very challenging at first but if you can get over the few times and stick to it, it is immensely rewarding.

Don't give up if you feel that the fasting plan you have chosen is too much for you. Ask your medical advisor to help you either modify your current plan or try another one. Not everyone is suited to each plan. You may find you need to try one or two before you are comfortable.

You don't have to dive right into adjusting your eating habits as well as try intermittent fasting all at once either. Start off fasting, eating normally but cutting down and gradually make food choice changes as you become more comfortable with fasting.

The trick is to find your balance, one step at a time if you must, as long as you are working to your end goal. How long it takes to get you there is entirely up to you. Don't think you have to rush headlong into it. Set achievable realistic goals that you feel one hundred percent comfortable with, otherwise your intermittent fasting diet is not going to work.

This is a lifestyle change, not a fad diet that you try for a few days or weeks and then forget because it became mundane or too challenging. This is a diet and lifestyle you need to commit to that will not only help you lose weight but be beneficial for your health. There is nothing wrong with easing into it; it is not a race and you have to remember you are doing this for you!

Well done on your decision to make a choice to try the intermittent fasting and all the very best. You can do this — you have got this!

References

9 Ways to Eat Clean. (2018, February 22). Retrieved from https://www.webmd.com/diet/ss/slideshow-how-to-eat-clean

Anapanasati. (n.d.). [PDF File] Retrieved from http://www.buddhanet.net/pdf_file/anapa-nasati.pdf

Arguin, H., Dionne, I. J., Sénéchal, M., Bouchard, D. R., Carpentier, A. C., Ardilouze, J.-L., ... Brochu, M. (2012, August). Short- and long-term effects of continuous versus intermittent restrictive diet approaches on body composition and the metabolic profile in overweight and obese postmenopausal women: a pilot study. Retrieved from https://www.ncbi.nlm.nih.gov/pubmed/22735163Barna, M. (2019, January 02). The science behind fasting diets. Retrieved from https://www.discovermagazine.com/health/fasting-may-be-more-than-a-fad-diet

Barnosky, A., Hoddy, K., Unterman, T. & Varady, K. (2014, October 01). Intermittent fasting vs daily calorie restriction for type 2 diabetes prevention: a review of human findings. Retrieved from https://www.sciencedirect.com/science/article/pii/S193152441400200X

Benefits of Intermittent Fasting for Women Over 50. (2019, September 03). Retrieved from https://prime-women.com/health/nutrition/benefits-of-intermittent-fasting-for-women-over-50/

Catterjee, S. (2016, January 01). Chapter two - Oxidative stress, inflammation, and disease. Retrieved from https://www.sciencedirect.com/science/article/pii/B9780128032695000024

Cole, W. (2017, November 09). The impact intermittent fasting can have on all your hormones. Retrieved from https://drwillcole.com/the-impact-intermittent-fasting-can-have-on-all-your-hormones/

Cronkleton, E. (2018, August 15). Taking a better breath. Retrieved from https://www.healthline.com/health/how-to-breathe

Dierks, T. (n.d.). Psychiatry research: Neuroimaging. Retrieved from https://www.journals.elsevier.com/psychiatry-research-neuroimaging/

Differential Effects of Alternate-Day Fasting Versus Daily Calorie Restriction on Insulin Resistance. (2019, September 27). Retrieved from https://www.ncbi.nlm.nih.gov/pubmed/31328895

Fasting — A History Part 1. (n.d.). Retrieved from https://thefastingmethod.com/fasting-a-history-part-i/

Fasting and Meditation: Everything You Need to Know. Retrieved from https://kenshoway.com/meditation/fasting-meditation-everything-you-need-to-know

Gunnars, K. (2018, July 25). Intermittent fasting 101 — The ultimate beginner's guide. Retrieved from https://www.healthline.com/nutrition/intermittent-fasting-guide

Hill, N. (1937). *Think and grow rich* (1937th ed.). Wise, Virginia: Napoleon Hill Foundation.

Hormones as you age. (n.d.). Retrieved from
https://www.rush.edu/health-wellness/discover-
health/hormones-you-age

LaBier, D. (2015, February 10). How meditation changes
the structure of your brain. Retrieved from
https://www.psychologytoday.com/us/blog/the-
new-resilience/201502/how-meditation-changes-
the-structure-your-brain

Holzel, B. K., CArmody, J., Vangel, M., Congleton, C., Yerramsetti, S. M., Gard, T., Lazar, S. W. (2011 January
30). Mindfulness practice leads to increases in re-
gional brain gray matter density. *Psychiatry Research: Neuroimaging*. Vol 191 (1) p36-43. Retrieved
from https://www.sciencedirect.com/science/arti-
cle/abs/pii/S092549271000288X

Papconstantinou, J. (2019, November 04). The role of sig-
naling pathways of inflammation and oxidative
stress in the development of senescence and aging
phenotypes in cardiovascular disease. Retrieved from
https://www.mdpi.com/2073-4409/8/11/1383

Rupasinghe, V. (2016, September 22). *Oxidative medicine
and cellular longevity* [PDF File]. Retrieved from
https://www.hindawi.com/jour-
nals/omcl/2016/7432797/

Shah, A. (n.d.). Intermittent Fasting Can Heal Your Gut &
Calm Inflammation. Here's Exactly How To Do It.
Retrieved from https://www.mindbodygreen.com/0-
28912/intermittent-fasting-can-heal-your-gut-calm-
inflammation-heres-exactly-how-to-it.html

The Health Benefits of Tai Chi. (2019, August 20). Retrieved from https://www.health.harvard.edu/stay-
ing-healthy/the-health-benefits-of-tai-chi

Valter, D. & Mattson, P. (2014, February 4). Fasting: Molecular Mechanisms and Clinical Applications. Retrieved from https://www.ncbi.nlm.nih.gov/pmc/articles/PMC3946160/

When Sciences Meets Mindfulness. (n.d.). Retrieved from https://news.harvard.edu/gazette/story/2018/04/harvard-researchers-study-how-mindfulness-may-change-the-brain-in-depressed-patients/

KETO DIET OVER 50

Ketogenic Diet for Senior Beginners & Weight Loss Book After 50.

Reset Your Metabolism with this Complete Guide for Women + 2 Weeks Meal Plan

**Dr. Gillian Keys Pomroy,
Dr. Anna Bernardi**

Introduction

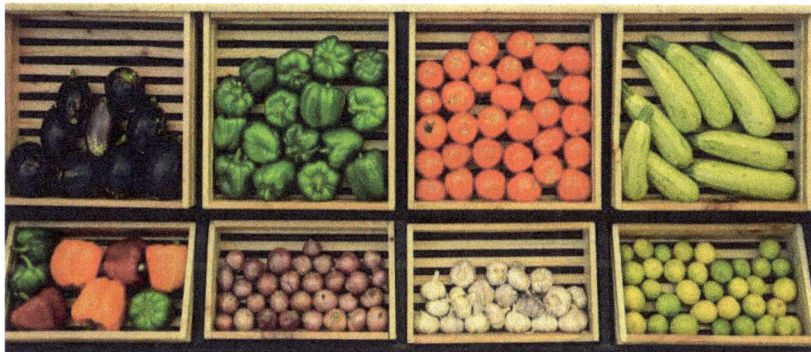

This is a beginner's guide to successfully maintaining a Keto diet, as a woman over the age of 50-years-old. Over the last few years, you have likely heard a lot about the Keto diet. It is known as being a diet that allows you to indulge, while still promoting weight loss. People of all ages have seen its incredible benefits.

Packed with foods that are rich in protein and high in fat and doing away with carbohydrates is the ultimate way that the Keto diet helps you to lose weight and maintain a healthy body. Instead of burning carbs, your body will be trained to burn fats, boosting your metabolism in an efficient way. It also turns your fats into ketones in your liver, which ends up providing you with additional energy for your brain.

Instead of focusing on the carbs that you will be giving up, the Keto diet aims its focus on all of the protein and fats that your body craves. Imaginably, there are many delicious recipes that you can follow and foods that you can eat, even when you aren't at home. The Keto diet is known for being one of the least restrictive diets; an important aspect in helping you to follow through with it. This guide will answer all of the questions that you have about what the diet consists of and how to successfully make Keto a part of your daily life. Unlike other diets, you will be amazed at how much freedom you are still allowed. It is almost like you aren't even on a diet at all!

As your body and brain ages, it is important to pay attention to all of the ways in which you can successfully maintain your energy levels. Certain tasks become a lot more cumbersome when you are running on half the energy than you're used to. The Keto diet works very well for women, especially those over 50. Aside from the benefits to your metabolism and energy levels, you will also notice a decrease in inflammation, a stable blood sugar level, and balanced hormones. With all of these benefits in place, you will notice that you will feel better both physically and mentally. And, of course, your mental health is very important to consider while on a diet. A lot of diets cause you to feel that you are lacking what you truly want to eat, therefore putting you into a negative mindset.

Keto is different and this guide will show you all of the reasons why. It is an overall lifestyle change that is possible for almost everyone, no matter what your average day looks like. You will be filled with plenty of optimism and all of the positivity necessary in order to meet your goals. Whether you want to maintain your current weight or lose weight in the process, Keto will help you get to where you truly want to be. It will become an anti-aging diet that will ultimately be a regular part of your everyday life.

You will experience all of these wonderful benefits as you begin your own Keto journey:

- Weight loss that lasts
- Lower blood sugar levels
- More energy
- Younger looking skin

- A boosted metabolism
- Balanced hormones
- Anti-aging benefits that work from the inside out
- A wide variety of delicious meals to eat

Most women can get the hang of Keto right away and experience few difficulties maintaining the diet. With the assistance of this guide, all of your questions about Keto will be fully answered.

If you are ready to feel great and look great, then you are ready to begin your own Keto diet. It will be a diet like no other because you will feel great every step of the way. There are no tricks or deceiving steps that you must take in order to succeed with the diet. As long as you are educated on what you need to be eating, you should have no problem incorporating the Keto diet into your current lifestyle. So, let's jump in and learn about the Keto diet, and how it can help you!

Chapter 1:
The History of the Ketogenic Diet: What is Keto?

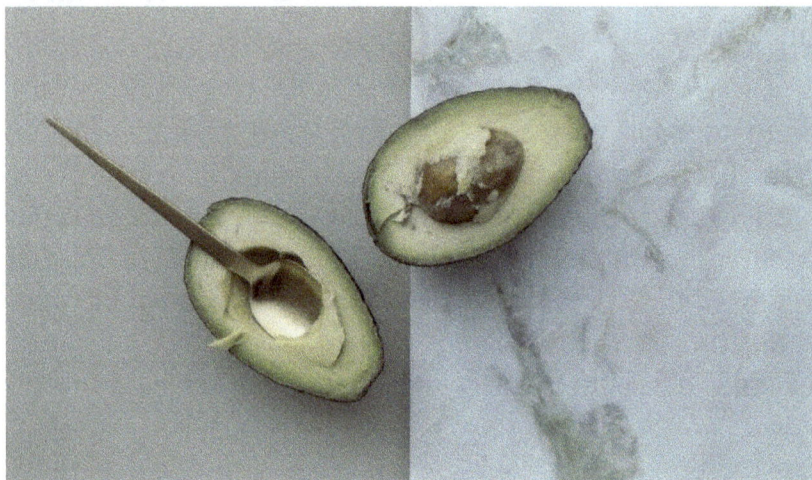

The Keto diet follows one basic principle — eliminate simple carbs and eat more fats in order to keep your body in a state of "fasting." When your body gets into this state, it will begin to burn ketones instead of burning glucose. Overall, this is thought to make you healthier without having to limit the quantity of food that you are eating on a daily basis.

Basically, the diet follows a model of 60-75% healthy fat consumption, 15-30% protein consumption, and only 5-10% carbs consumption, in order to change the way that you process energy. A lot of people are skeptical at first because it seems like it is a diet with minimal rules; but it truly is that simple.

Putting your body into a state of ketosis is ultimately your main goal. Your system normally chooses to run on glucose, which is sugar. When you eliminate the consumption of carbs, this causes your body to think that it is "starving," but you won't feel that way. From this point, your body will make the necessary adjustments that it needs to make in order to shift its focus. It will then generate a secondary source of energy that is derived from fat in order to keep the glucose flowing to the brain. Without the presence of so many carbs, your body will break down all of the fat compounds into ketones; an alternative fuel source.

Many people have realized that following this diet provides impressive results. Not only will your weight be properly managed, but you will also end up feeling healthier and more energized than ever before. The term "ketogenic" is fairly new, only being used since the 20th century. But even before this term was introduced, the Ancient Greeks were big advocates for restricting diets in order to treat diseases such as epilepsy. An interesting history, indeed, that deserves a quick exploration.

Back in the days of Hippocrates, fasting was the only known treatment for epilepsy. This became a very standard practice over the next two thousand years. It began to spread from Europe throughout the whole world. While today, most people utilize the Keto diet to manage their weight and health, its origins very clearly state that it was meant to reprogram the brain. Epileptic patients in 1911 were recorded having fewer seizures and fewer epilepsy symptoms while on a Keto diet versus being on a regular diet. It only took a few periods of regular fasting for them to see these results.

It was around the same time in the United States that an osteopathic physician, Hugh Conklin, started to recommend fasting as a treatment method for his epileptic patients. They would fast for 18-25 days at a time, and the success rates were incredible. Most patients reported that they experienced a 50% success rate, for adults, and a whopping 90% success rate for children. Of course, this is an extreme version of the now-refined diet that we know about today. While the results were very impressive, health professionals knew that this wasn't a permanent solution. Fasting is inherently temporary. Once the patients returned to their normal diets, the seizures would come back just as quickly.

Once this problem became apparent, doctors got to work in order to modify the treatment plan into one that could become long-lasting. Instead of restricting all calories equally, doctors began focusing on eliminating only certain sugars and starches to study these effects. Dr. Wilder at the Mayo Clinic was a well-known physician who took part in the studies. He noticed right away that his patients were having fewer seizures with their lower blood sugar levels. Dr. Wilder was responsible for officially creating the Keto diet as a lifestyle instead of merely a temporary treatment plan. The diet that we are all familiar with now mimics the way that your metabolism reacts during a period of fasting.

A simple concept evolved into a simple diet plan. Patients were able to stay in a permanent state of fasting without actually feeling that they were starving themselves. This shift in what you consume triggers your body to automatically receive the benefits of the ketones. This allowed people to feel that they were still getting all of the calories and nutrition that they needed but tricked the body into metabolizing as if they were starving. It was a fascinating discovery that truly shaped the Keto diet into what it is today.

Another Mayo Clinic physician, Dr. M.G. Peterman was credited for standardizing the diet. He called it the "classic keto" approach. This is an approach that is often still used today. A 4:1 ratio of fat to protein and carbs must be maintained. 90% of all calories come from fat, while 6% come from protein and only 4% from carbs. This is often thought of as an ideal approach to the Keto diet, while a 3:1 ratio is also considered highly beneficial. This might sound extreme on paper, but it truly isn't hard to maintain because your body still recognizes that it is getting all of the nutrition that it needs.

There is typically one big question that remains after reading about the Keto diet, and that involves what you can actually eat. Historically, the following foods were known as essentials while being on the diet:

- Vegetables without Starch: broccoli, cauliflower, cabbage, leafy greens, onions, and peppers
- Full Fat Dairy: Cheese, yogurt, and milk
- Protein: eggs, soybeans, shellfish, fish, pork, poultry, and beef
- Nuts and Seeds: almonds, pistachios, walnuts, sunflower seeds, and pumpkin seeds
- Quality Fats: unlimited from both plant and animal sources
- Fruits (sparingly): avocado, rhubarb, coconut, and berries

Doctors would put emphasis on using precise measurements in order to achieve the maximum results. These ratios would be followed very carefully. It became so precise that the food was measured to the gram before each patient was able to consume it. The medical professionals could now see that this diet that mimicked fasting could be maintained for far longer periods of time.

Now, two centuries later the Keto diet has remained fairly unchanged. Nutritionists have created guidelines that suggest participants consume one gram of protein per kilogram of body weight. 10-15 grams of carbohydrates are acceptable, with the rest of the diet being focused on eating fats.

Scientifically, it is still hard to explain why the Keto diet is and was so successful for epileptics. The main theory that has been created states that the ketones' natural structures cause them to have an anti-electrical response in the brain. This means that people who experience seizures are no longer being exposed to these electrical currents, therefore preventing future seizures from occurring. It is fascinating to think about its results regarding epileptic patients, but the benefits are not limited. It didn't take much time for doctors to realize that the Keto diet could also benefit those who were not epileptic.

Interestingly enough, this discovery came when the diet was tested on children. The children who were put on the diet were noted as being less irritable, more focused, and easier to discipline. They were also to get better sleep at night, further benefiting them. Follow up research has since been done in the 2000s and it showed the same results. With the development of anticonvulsant drugs, the eating strategy was pushed aside. The Keto diet only recently resurfaced as a valid diet plan and lifestyle choice.

During this time when the Keto approach was being set aside, it lost a lot of momentum. This caused people to use it incorrectly, not following its precise measurements. Fewer dieticians were experienced with the diet and did not know how to properly coach their patients through it. Because of these bad experiences, people saw the Keto diet as something negative and ineffective. In just a matter of decades, the Keto diet had a bad stigma attached to it that prevented people from wanting to experience it. This marked a time period of the initial disappearance of the Keto diet, used as a treatment plan or diet plan.

Revisiting Keto

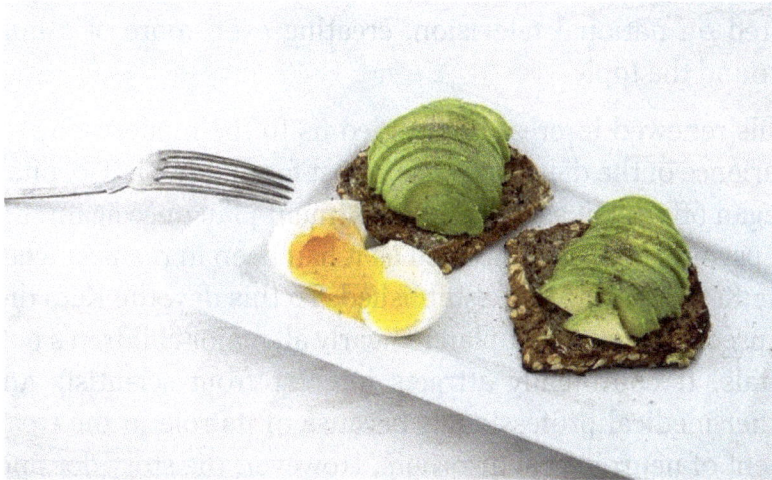

Keto returned to the mainstream in the 1990s. Those who were still interested in it studied it because of its mysterious workings rather than as a diet plan to follow. This went on for the next several years until an episode of the news television program Dateline, in 1994, shed some positive light on Keto.

In the episode, a 2-year-old child was featured. He had been experiencing severe epilepsy. His seizures were out of control until he was placed on the Keto diet. It was a risky move, but his doctors at John Hopkins did not know what else to try. The severity of his disorder led them down the Keto path. At this time, fewer than 10 children were being treated in this way for epilepsy each year.

After the show aired, it triggered a major response from medical professionals and regular people alike. Not to mention, a huge increase in scientific interest. All of the gears began turning again as people took interest in the Keto diet once again. It even led to the creation of a film called "First Do No Harm," created by this child's father. Released in 1997, the movie starred Meryl Streep and revolves around the experience of with the diet and how much it helped their child. It aired on national television, creating even more of a buzz around the topic.

This renewed interest in Keto led us to the modern-day experience of the diet that we are most familiar with. Hospitals began offering it as a reliable treatment plan once again. Epilepsy was now being treated as it had been in the past when the Keto diet was first established. To this day, the Keto diet is used as a treatment plan in nearly all major children's hospitals. It continually attracts interest from scientists and other medical professionals because of its role in the treatment of neurological disorders. However, the story does not end there.

If the Keto diet were only beneficial to those who were experiencing epilepsy, its interest may have died down by now. Since the diet has been back in the spotlight, a lot of people have realized how beneficial it is for controlling physical health and weight management. Once this perspective of the Keto diet shifted, it gained a lot of attention from those wishing to live a healthier lifestyle. This renewed interest in Keto allowed researchers to see that it could be used as solely a diet plan, even for those who were completely neurologically healthy.

It took additional time for Keto to really become a trustworthy diet plan that is used by people who do not have epilepsy. While it was regaining momentum in the 90s, so was the Atkins diet. If you have been following diet trends for the last few decades, you likely already know what Atkins entails. This diet plan has a similar outlook when it comes to carbs and the way it was presented really took off during this time. Though Atkins dominated the spotlight, this allowed even more room for scientists and researchers to take Keto seriously as a standalone diet plan. The two were compared to each other often in the late 90s, making room for the diet that we now know so much about.

In today's society, Atkins has slowly faded away to make room for Keto. A lot of people found Atkins to be too strict and complicated. Eating out or away from home was a challenge for those partaking in the diet plan. Keto aimed to change this perspective. It proved to people that they can still lose weight and maintain a satisfying lifestyle while doing so. Many would argue that being on Keto does not feel like a diet plan at all. Instead, it acts as a guideline for how we need to treat our bodies by providing a method that is simple yet effective. Keto is so enjoyable because it doesn't ask you to count calories every single day. It is a more flexible diet plan that allows individuals to still feel that they are individuals.

Aside from proving itself to nutritionists and people alike, Keto is thriving in a time where social media is very popular. As people go through their Keto journeys, it is easy to access this real-time progress in a way that feels comforting and informative. On any given social media platform, it is not usual to see that people are posting about their experience with the Keto diet. Along with this praise, people also love to post pictures of their food! While the early 2000s gave us a lot more freedom of information thanks to the internet, this current decade allows us to dive even deeper. Seeing these real experiences that people are having with Keto makes it more relatable. It also gives us ideas for recipes and how the Keto diet can be enjoyed.

The message remains simple to this day — pay attention to how your body feels. Starting any new diet plan can be questionable, especially if you do not know exactly how to execute it and apply it to your own life. The findings behind the Keto diet continue to impress those of varying backgrounds and in different geographical locations. When first starting your own Keto journey, your body is going to feel different immediately. This is because of what is actually going on internally. Unlike many other gimmick diets or fads, Keto doesn't promise rapid or unrealistic weight loss. Instead, it provides an overall lifestyle solution that can be followed by anyone.

Whether you are still on the fence about starting your own Keto journey or you have all of the resources that you need, the results will speak for themselves. Naturally, our bodies weaken as we age. This can send us into a frenzy of trying the latest health crazes and forcing us to eat foods that we don't really enjoy. Being open-minded about Keto is important in the beginning. As long as you are listening to your body, keeping your portions similar to what you are used to eating, and being creative with your meals, you will find that the Keto journey can be a wonderful addition to your life.

As a woman over 50, you have an awareness about your overall health that you probably didn't have when you were younger. And, that's natural. The purpose of this book is to help you bring that awareness into action - specifically tapping into the benefits of the Keto diet. While it's a relatively easy change to make in your life, there are things you need to know before you dive in, that we'll be covering throughout this book. First and foremost, the different types and strategies of ketogenic diets. So, we'll start there next.

Chapter 2:
Types of Ketogenic: SKD, TKD, and CKD

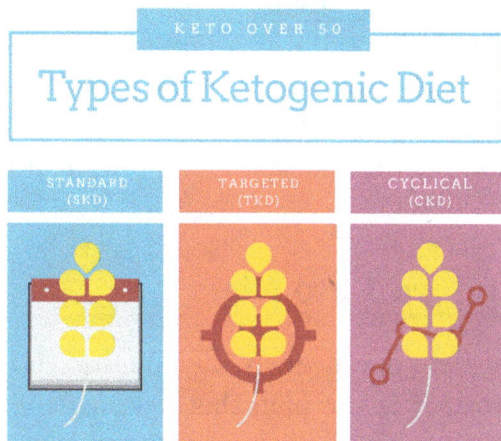

KETO OVER 50

Types of Ketogenic Diet

STANDARD (SKD)   TARGETED (TKD)   CYCLICAL (CKD)

Having flexibility with your diet plan is a significant positive factor in being able to stick with it. While you now have a basic understanding of how Keto came to be, there is also more information to delve into by researching the various types of the diet that you can follow. If you do not want to take a standard approach, know that you do have options.

Keto actually allows you to modify the diet in three different ways depending on what you currently need. This gives you even more freedom to feel great and to feel like you are not on a diet at all. Most other diet plans do not have these options, making them seem stricter. Keto aims to give everyone a plan that works for them, not just a single template that must be followed.

The difference between these forms of Keto comes in the percentages of the foods that you will be eating. While they all believe in the core concept of eliminating carbs in order to get your body into ketosis, there are many ways that this can be done. For example, if you are imagining a breadless diet that will leave you feeling cranky all the time, you will be pleased to find that there are forms of the diet that allow you to have carbs during certain times. You might find that you will try all three forms of the diet in order to see which one works best for you. Depending on what you are used to eating already, this is likely going to shape the decision that you make. It is great because switching between these three variations is not extreme or dangerous. They vary just enough to give you options without sacrificing your health in the process.

SKD: Standard Keto Diet

The standard Keto diet is likely the one that you have heard about the most. It is the plan that people generally like to start with because it provides a great foundation and introduction to the lifestyle. This diet involves a low-carb and moderate-protein approach. The focus is on maintaining a high-fat meal plan.

An example of the SKD includes the individual eating 75% fat, 20% protein, and 5% carbs. (This is the general guideline that you will follow each day.) People enjoy this method because it does not change; these simple principles are relatively easy to maintain once you get used to them. The SKD has been studied the most extensively. When you read about Keto, it is likely the SKD method that researchers are referring to.

A summary of its benefits includes effective weight loss. For most, this is one of the biggest concerns when starting any diet plan. If you feel that you want to lose weight safely, the SKD will allow you to do so in a healthy way. The reason why this works so well is that you never experience periods of intense hunger like you would with other diets. At no point in time should you feel that you are truly starving yourself when you are on the Keto diet. This feeling will only lead to negative results because the body will want to stray from the plan. You've probably experienced this first-hand while trying other diets. When you are hungry enough, you lose motivation and are more prone to eat unhealthy foods that tend to "comfort" you. Losing progress in this way can become very discouraging.

Another benefit of being on the SKD is that your risk factor for diseases and ailments will be lowered. Giving you a well-rounded meal plan, Keto aims to push you in a healthy direction that you can easily take. Because you won't be consumed with counting calories or limiting your food intake, you will be able to fully appreciate this benefit while you are on the diet. Keto feels so great because it is a lot different than a low-fat diet. Since your body is still getting plenty of protein, you will be less likely to stray. One study has actually found that being on the Keto diet has shown a success rate with weight loss that is up to 2.2 times more effective than other similar diets.

Your risk factor for diabetes should be taken into account when starting the Keto diet. As you age, this risk factor can naturally increase. Two of the biggest problems have to do with a change in metabolism and a spike in your blood sugar. As you know, the SKD places a lot of focus on redirecting your metabolism and keeping your blood sugar down. While being on the Keto diet, you are going to be losing weight due to your body burning the bad fats that aren't necessary to its functionality. In turn, it will be getting rid of the excess fats that you do not need. This is another way that Keto can greatly benefit someone who is pre-diabetic or has a genetic history of diabetes.

The benefits do not end there. The SKD has been known for reducing your risk of cancer, heart disease, Alzheimer's, and polycystic ovary syndrome. With aging comes increased risks in many or all of these conditions. It is impressive to think that Keto can provide comprehensive benefits; enough to protect you from all of these diseases. By not giving up all of the foods that you love, you will feel great about your journey.

Keeping in mind that Keto is not only effective but preventative, may increase your motivation as you plan out your meals and figure out what other aspects of your life must be changed in order to adjust the way you are eating. It isn't hard to remember what to do while on Keto. As long as you are staying away from sugary foods, both natural and artificial, you are allowing your body to adjust to the diet naturally. Placing a focus on making meat and dairy taste delicious, you won't even notice the carbs that you are replacing.

TKD: Targeted Keto Diet

The targeted Keto diet focuses on workout plans that you have in place. While you know that sticking to a healthy diet is very important, another aspect of this is your effort placed on exercising and getting up and moving. The main difference between the TKD and the SKD is that you will actually be consuming carbs before you work out. This will provide you with a boost of energy when you need it most, allowing you to focus on your physical fitness. The amount of exercise that you are doing needs to increase and be modified as you age. You likely can't do the things that you used to do when you were younger, but that doesn't mean that physical fitness needs to be put in the background. Staying very much in the foreground, taking part in the TKD means that you need to have a solid fitness routine.

In order to make this plan work for you, it takes a little bit of preparation before you actually begin to change your eating habits. Think about the exercises that you enjoy doing and that are suitable for your current level of physical fitness. While there is always room for growth and an increase in intensity, you need to start with something basic in order to not overdo it. Starting with light to moderate exercise twice weekly, you will be able to begin building your diet around your fitness routine. The principle is simple — eat Keto for five days out of the week and then eat carbs on the two days that you intend on getting your exercise in. This plan is for those who intend on keeping up with a regular fitness routine. It will show you adverse effects if you eat based on the TKD method without including exercise in the plan.

You can still have a fat loss goal while following the TKD plan. What is essential to remember is that you do not overeat on your days of carb-consumption. Since you are going to be allowing your body carbs selectively, you need to remember that these carbs are going to count as calories. Because of this, you also need to adjust the number of fats that you are eating on those days. It all needs to balance itself out and this can be the trickiest part of getting the hang of the TKD. Only you can hold yourself accountable for how much exercise you plan on completing and how many carbs you plan on eating. It can take some trial and error to get this ratio right, but that is normal.

The TKD is a middle ground between the SKD and the CKD. It allows you to perform at a high intensity for short periods of time without taking your body out of ketosis for too long. For many, the TKD has been shown to build up endurance and allow you to truly evolve with your physical fitness goals. This plan is most appropriate for those who are beginner-intermediate level with the Keto diet. If this sounds like something that can be incorporated into your lifestyle, you will find many benefits to this targeted approach. It allows you to aim higher with your fitness goals, showing you yet another reason how the Keto diet is not a diet filled with limitations or strictness.

Over time, exercise is going to feel less strenuous. When you get to this point, it is a good idea to revisit your fitness plan to see if it is still suitable for you. While it isn't great to change your diet frequently, you can safely adjust the TKD if you feel that you are ready to move up to more intense physical activity. Know that this is simply an option that it provides. You do not have to change anything if you feel that your body is doing well and that you are maintaining growth in your endurance. It is best to stick with your diet for at least a month before altering it too much. When you do consume your carbs, it is best to do so 30 minutes prior to exercising. Many people find that 25-50 grams of carbs are the right amount to allow them to power through their workouts.

CKD: Cyclical Keto Diet

As implied earlier, the CKD method is going to be the form of Keto that fluctuates the most. This diet plan involves a rotation that has you switching from the traditional high-fat, low-carb regimen to one that allows for higher carb intake. Of all the types of Keto, this one involves the most structure and guidelines. In the CKD, you are going to allow your body "refeeding days." This means that you will select a few days each week where you eat higher amounts of carbs in order to replenish your body's glucose levels. People choose to follow the CKD when they are focusing on muscle growth. Bodybuilders and those who are more serious about working out tend to follow this plan, for instance. Be aware, however, of all the types of Keto that are followed today, the CKD has the least amount of research to back it.

Many people confuse the CKD with carb cycling, but the two are different. When you are carb cycling, you follow a similar structure of cutting carbs on some days and then replenishing your body with carbs on the other days. The week is usually divided by 4-6 days of lower carb intake and 1-3 days of higher carb intake. One main difference between carb cycling and the CKD is that the former does not allow you to reach a state of ketosis. This means that you are not going to be getting all of the benefits that Keto has to offer.

This plan is likely going to be least applicable to you, but it is still important to learn about it, as it is still a viable form of Keto that many follows. Basically, on standard days, the individual must consume fewer than 50 grams of carbs each day. Healthy fats should make up approximately 75% of the diet. Some options include avocados, eggs, dairy products, nut butters, and fatty meats. Protein makes up about 15-20% of this diet. On refeeding days, you can consume carbs in a larger amount. Carbs will actually make up about 60-70% of your total calories, with protein making up 15-20% and fats 5-10%. As you can see, there is a big fluctuation between standard days and refeeding days.

A common misconception is that those on the CKD eat a lot of bread in order to get their carbs on refeeding days. But, that's not the typical, or healthy recommendation. Generally, the CKD method means that the extra carbs come from healthier sources, like sweet potatoes, butternut squash, brown rice, quinoa, oats, and other whole-grain foods. As you can see, there is still discipline required on those days, even despite the spike in carb intake. All of these carbs are very high in vitamins and nutrients. Foods and drinks that are sugary and artificial are still avoided because they simply lack any valuable nutrients. If you are not planning on pairing your diet with a relatively intense workout plan and routine, the CKD is likely not going to be the diet that works for you.

We also suggest that you incorporate some intermittent fasting when following the CKD. This means that, after your refeeding days, you fast for a few hours at a time. This will get you back to ketosis quicker. Your workouts should be done following your refeeding days to take full advantage of ketosis and to get into a prime condition for muscle growth. Those who wish to follow the diet for simple weight management or anti-aging will not get any additional benefits by following the CKD because it is simply an intensified version of Keto. However, you can benefit from CKD if you regularly partake in high-intensity workouts on a weekly basis or are planning on incorporating that level of activity in your life.

The main benefit of the CKD method is the potential for muscle growth and endurance-building abilities when it comes to sports or other athletic activities. One downside is that people often complain of constipation while on the CKD because of the fluctuating refeeding days. In order to combat this, it is important to watch your fiber intake, and make sure to hydrate accordingly. The CKD is a big commitment when it comes to dieting and it is advised that you try to maintain the SKD for several months, before you transition into the CKD.

Whichever plan you select, SKD, TKD or CKD, will depend on your current state of health as well as your health goals. The bottom line is that the Keto diet can work for people who have a wide variety of needs and aspirations. But, why is the Keto diet perfect for women over 50? Let's explore that, next.

Chapter 3:
Why Women Over 50?

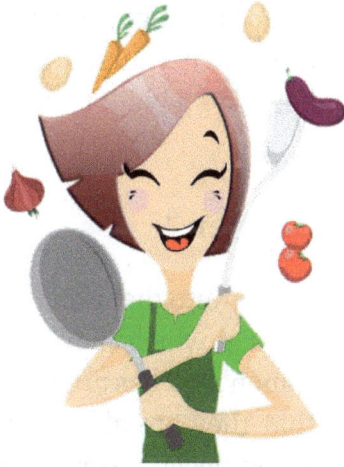

As a woman, you have likely experienced significant differences in the way that you must diet compared to the way that men can diet. Women tend to have a harder time losing weight because of their different hormones and the way their bodies break down fats. Another factor to consider is your age group. As the body ages, it is important to be more attentive with the way that you care for yourself. Aging bodies start to experience problems more quickly and this can be avoided with the proper diet and exercise plan. Keto works well for women of all ages and this is because of how it communicates with the body. No matter how fit you are right now or how much weight you need or want to lose, Keto is going to change the way that your body metabolizes, giving you a very personalized experience.

When starting your Keto diet, you should not be thinking about extremes because that isn't what Keto should be about.

You should be able to place your body into ketosis without feeling terrible in the process. One of the biggest guidelines to follow while starting your Keto journey is that you need to listen to your body regularly. If you ever feel that you are starving or simply unfulfilled, then you will likely have to modify the way you are eating because it isn't reaching ketosis properly. It is not an overnight journey, so you need to remember to be patient with yourself and with your body. Adapting to a Keto diet takes a bit of transition time and a lot of awareness.

Why Keto for Women?

The health benefits of the Keto diet are not different for men or women, but the speed at which they are reached does differ. As mentioned, women's bodies are a lot different when it comes to the ways that they are able to burn fats and lose weight. For example, by design women have at least 10% more body fat than men. No matter how fit you are, this is just an aspect of being a woman that you must consider. Don't be hard on yourself if you notice that it seems like men can lose weight easier — that's because they can! What women have in additional body fat, men typically have the same in muscle mass. This is why men tend to see faster external results, because that added muscle mass means that their metabolism rates are higher. That increased metabolism means that fat and energy get burned faster. When you are on Keto, though, the internal change is happening right away.

Your metabolism is unique, but it is also going to be slower than a man's by nature. Since muscle is able to burn more calories than fat, the weight just seems to fall off of men, giving them the ability to reach the opportunity for muscle growth quickly. This should not be something that holds you back from starting your Keto journey. As long as you are keeping these realistic bodily factors in mind, you won't be left wondering why it is taking you a little bit longer to start losing weight. This point will come for you, but it will take a little bit more of a process that you must be committed to following through with.

Another unique condition that a woman can experience but a man cannot be PCOS or Polycystic Ovary Syndrome; a hormonal imbalance that causes the development of cysts. These cysts can cause pain, interfere with normal reproductive function, and, in extreme and dangerous cases, burst. PCOS is actually very common among women, affecting up to 10% of the entire female population. Surprisingly, most women are not even aware that they have the condition. Around 70% of women have PCOS that is undiagnosed. This condition can cause a significant hormonal imbalance, therefore affecting your metabolism. It can also inevitably lead to weight gain, making it even harder to see results while following diet plans. In order to stay on top of your health, you must make sure that you are going to the gynecologist regularly.

Menopause is another reality that must be faced by women, especially as we age. Most women begin the process of menopause in their mid-40s. Men do not go through menopause, so they are spared from yet another condition that causes slower metabolism and weight gain. When you start menopause, it is easy to gain weight and lose muscle. Most women, once menopause begins, lose muscle at a much faster rate, and conversely gain weight, despite dieting and exercise regimens. Keto can, therefore, be the right diet plan for you. Regardless of what your body is doing naturally, via processes like menopause, your internal systems are still going to be making the switch from running on carbs to deriving energy from fats.

When the body begins to successfully run on fats, you have an automatic fuel reserve waiting to be burned. It will take some time for your body to do this, but when it does, you will actually be able to eat fewer calories and still feel just as full because your body knows to take energy from the fat that you already have. This will become automatic. It is, however, a process that requires some patience, but being aware of what is actually going on with your body can help you stay motivated while on Keto.

Because a Keto diet reduces the amount of sugar you are consuming, it naturally lowers the amount of insulin in your bloodstream. This can actually have amazing effects on any existing PCOS and fertility issues, as well as menopausal symptoms and conditions like pre-diabetes and Type 2 diabetes. Once your body adjusts to a Keto diet, you are overcoming the things that are naturally in place that can be preventing you from losing weight and getting healthy. Even if you placed your body on a strict diet, if it isn't getting rid of sugars properly, you likely aren't going to see the same results that you will when you try Keto. This is a big reason why Keto can be so beneficial for women.

As we've discussed, carbs and sugar can have a huge impact on your hormonal balance. You might not even realize that your hormones are not in balance until you experience a lifestyle that limits carbs and eliminates sugars. Keto is going to reset this balance for you, keeping your hormones at healthy levels. As a result of this, you will probably find yourself in a better general mood, and with much more energy to get through your days.

For women over 50, there are guidelines to follow when you start your Keto diet. As long as you are following the method properly and listening to what your body truly needs, you should have no more problems than men do while following the plan. What you will have are more obstacles to overcome, but you can do it. Remember that plenty of women successfully follow a Keto diet and see great results. Use these women as inspiration for how you anticipate your own journey to go. On the days when it seems impossible, remember what you have working against you, but more importantly what you have working for you. Your body is designed to go into ketogenesis more than it is designed to store fat by overeating carbs. Use this as a motivation to keep pushing you ahead. Keto is a valid option for you and the results will prove this, especially if you are over the age of 50.

Why Keto for 50+?

As we age, we naturally look for ways to hold onto our youth and energy. It's not uncommon to think about things that promote anti-aging. Products and lifestyle changes are advertised everywhere, and they are designed to catch your attention, as you grapple with the reality of what it means to be a 50+ year-old woman in our society. Even if you aren't eating for the purposes of anti-aging yet, you have likely thought about it in terms of the way you treat your skin and hair, for example. The great thing about the Keto diet is that it supports maximum health, from the inside out; working hard to make sure that you are in the best shape that you can be in.

For instance, indigestion becomes common as you age. This happens because the body is not able to break down certain foods as well as it used to. With all of the additives and fillers, we all become used to putting our bodies through discomfort in an attempt to digest regular meals. You are probably not even aware that you are doing this to your body, but upon trying a Keto diet, you will realize how your digestion will begin to change. You will no longer feel bloated or uncomfortable after you eat. If you notice this as a common feeling, you are likely not eating food that is nutritious enough to satisfy your needs and is only resulting in excess calories.

Keto fills you up in all of the ways that you need, allowing your body to truly digest and metabolize all of the nutrients. When you eat your meals, you should not feel the need to overeat in order to overcompensate for not having enough nutrients. Anything that takes stress off of any system in your body is going to become a form of anti-aging. You will quickly find this benefit once you start your Keto journey, as it is one of the first-reported changes that most participants notice. In addition to a healthier digestive system, you will also experience more regular bathroom usage, with little to none of the problems often associated with age.

While weight loss is one of the more common desires for most 50+ women who start a diet plan, the way that the weight is lost matters. If you have ever shed a lot of weight before, you have probably experienced the adverse effects of sagging or drooping skin that you were left to deal with. Keto actually rejuvenates the elasticity in your skin. This means that you will be able to lose weight and your skin will be able to catch up. Instead of having to do copious amounts of exercise to firm up your skin, it should already be becoming firmer each day that you are on the Keto diet. This is something that a lot of participants are pleasantly surprised to find out.

Women also commonly report a natural reduction in wrinkles, and healthier skin and hair growth, in general. Many women who start the diet report that they actually notice reverse effects in their aging process. While the skin becomes healthier and more supple, it also becomes firmer. Even if you aren't presently losing weight, you will still be able to appreciate the effects that Keto brings to your skin and face. Because your internal systems are becoming healthier by the day, this tends to show on the outside in a short amount of time. You will also begin to feel healthier. While it is possible to read about the experiences of others, there is nothing like feeling this for yourself when you begin Keto.

Everyone, especially women over 50, has day-to-day tasks that are draining and require certain amounts of energy to complete. Aging can, unfortunately, take away from your energy reserve, even if you get enough sleep at night. It limits the way that you have to live your life, and this can become a very frustrating realization. Most diet plans bring about a sluggish feeling that you are simply supposed to get used to, for example. But Keto does the exact opposite. When you change your eating habits to fit the Keto guidelines, you are going to be hit with a boost of energy. Since your body is truly getting everything that it needs nutritionally, it will repay you with a sustained energy supply.

Another common complaint for women over 50 is that, seemingly overnight, your blood sugar levels are going to be more sensitive than usual. While it is important that everyone keeps an eye on these levels, it is especially important for those who are in their 50s and beyond. High blood sugar can be an indication that diabetes is on the way, but Keto can become a preventative measure, that we've already talked about. Additionally, naturally regulating elevated blood sugar levels, also reduces systemic inflammation, which is also common for women over 50. By balancing the immune system, of which inflammation is a part of, common aches and pains are reduced. If, for example, you've noticed that you have been feeling stiff lately, even despite your efforts to exercise and stretching, this is likely due to a normal case of inflamed joints. Inflammation can also affect vital organs and is a precursor to cancer. Keto will support your path to an anti-inflammatory lifestyle.

Sugar is never great for us, but it turns out that sugar can become especially dangerous as we age. What is known as a "sugar sag" can occur when you get older because the excess sugar molecules will attach themselves to skin and protein in your body. This doesn't even necessarily happen because you are eating too much sugar. Average levels of sugar intake can also lead to this sagging as the sugar weakens the strength of your proteins that are supposed to hold you together. With sagging comes even more wrinkles and arterial stiffening.

If you have any anti-aging concerns, the Keto diet will likely be able to address your worries. It is a diet that works extremely hard while allowing you a fairly simple and direct guideline to follow in return. While your motivation is necessary in order to form a successful relationship with Keto, you won't need to worry about doing anything "wrong" or accidentally breaking from your diet. As long as you know how to give up your sugary foods and drinks while making sure that you are consuming the correct amount of carbs, you will be able to find your own success while on the diet.

As a woman over 50, you'll find that you will feel better, healthier and younger, by implementing the simple steps that will tune your body into processing excess fats for energy. You'll build muscle, lose fat, and look and feel younger. As we've touched on, a Keto diet helps balance your hormones, reversing and/or eliminating many common menopausal signs and symptoms. Let's explore how, in the next chapter.

Chapter 4:
Balance Hormones and Boost Energy

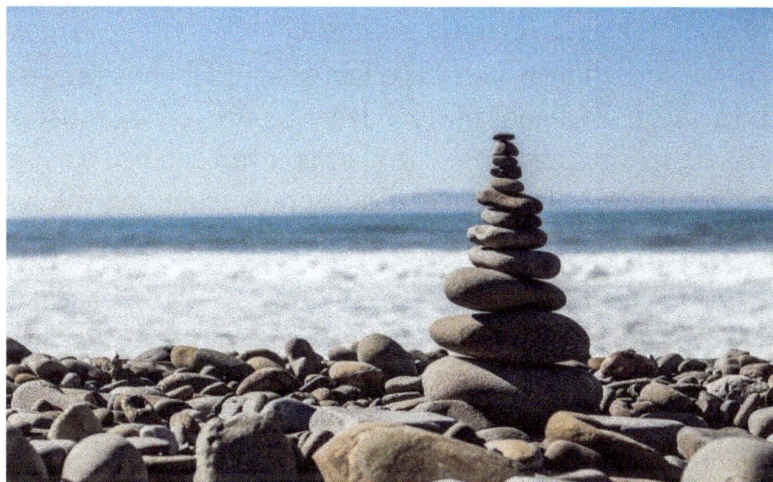

In the previous chapter, you learned a little bit about the ways in which Keto can provide great benefits for your hormones and energy levels. Considering how much you rely on both of these things each day, this is going to allow you to feel great while you are on the diet. There is nothing worse than starting a diet to find that it drags you down. Keto, when done correctly, will not make you feel this way. You will know that you are doing everything you need to do when you see that your energy is increasing. All of your hormones will also begin to balance out. This can leave you feeling naturally happier and calmer in your daily life.

If you have been experiencing difficulty with balancing your hormones, especially if you are going through menopause, you know how cumbersome these side effects can be. From hot flashes to mood swings, you have likely experienced it all in a very short period of time. This can become very discouraging because it can often feel that nothing helps the symptoms. Many women who are presently going through this have started to try Keto as a desperate attempt to make a difference and they are finding that it does, indeed, help level things out. Even if your symptoms are very bad, Keto has been shown to lessen them and make your life feel easier again.

It works so well because of the increase in fat consumption. While you have likely never been encouraged to consume *more* fat in any previous diet plan you've been on, Keto allows you to do this because it is literally changing the way that your body stores and breaks down this fat. When your body has more of these good fats inside, it will be prompted to create more estrogen and progesterone. This shows that, when you start a diet that slashes your fat consumption, you might actually be causing this hormonal imbalance to become more severe without even realizing it.

For those still dealing with periods, Keto helps by detoxifying the body. PMS symptoms are lessened when the body reaches this point of detoxification. PMS can become very hard to deal with because it produces an excess of estrogen. When you have too much estrogen in your system, this is when you will begin to feel cramping, bloating, and mood swings that you have been dealing with for years. This estrogen dominance can occur more severely in certain cases when your diet consists of too many sugary foods. What you need is additional progesterone in order to balance you out. Because the Keto diet detoxifies you, it will be getting rid of the excess hormones that you don't need and begin to replace them with the ones that you are lacking.

As discussed, many women struggle with PCOS without even realizing it. While fertility might no longer be an issue for you, PCOS still brings forth many unpleasant side effects as you age. Because there is no cure for it, management of the disorder is essential. If you suffer from PCOS, poor blood sugar regulation and excess body fat can be making this a lot worse. Keto has been seen as a viable solution for easing the stress of PCOS. During a Duke University study, everyone who followed the diet found that they were able to lose weight and those seeking improvement with fertility were actually able to become healthy enough to get pregnant.

Insulin is a very big hormone that is important to your body. This controls your blood sugar and when this gets too low, can also begin to impact your sex hormone levels. What Keto does to your body is makes it more insulin sensitive. With a balanced level of insulin in your body, this will mean that your cells are going to use it properly. Studies have found that up to 75% of obese patients with diabetes experienced this positive increase in insulin sensitivity. An impressive number, these results appear very promising. While being more insulin sensitive, you are also able to get fit more easily. Any weight you lose will be easier to keep off. This, in turn, lowers your risk for cardiovascular disease and dementia.

An instant way to feel depleted is by having to deal with copious amounts of stress with no relief. When you are handling the stressors in your daily life, your adrenal glands will begin to release cortisol in order to keep up with what is going on. This is your body's attempt at providing you with extra energy to handle the tough situations that you face. This can become a problem though, because your body can actually begin to produce too much cortisol. It also robs your body of the necessary estrogen and progesterone that it seeks.

While your body thinks that it is helping your stress by giving you this cortisol, it is actually detrimental to your sexual health, your muscle mass, and your overall point of burnout. The body is more fragile when it is in this heightened state and Keto aims to provide you with a more balanced approach. No one enjoys feeling like they just can't make it through their days, so it is best that you do not let your body overcompensate for what it mistakenly thinks that you need. The Keto diet will redirect it and guide you in the right direction.

You will notice that there is a pattern present — fewer fats in your diet equals fewer results. Most diet plans like to focus on cutting out these fats and this is what makes Keto so unique. It seems like a reasonable request to cut out fats, but when your body is left with only carbs and sugars to digest, this is actually going to be detrimental to your weight loss, your overall health and it is going to throw off your hormones. Many people come to this realization after tirelessly trying diet after diet. The Keto plan is designed to be your end-all plan, one that can work with you for the rest of your life.

Tired of Being Tired

If feeling worn out seems to be a regular pattern in your life nowadays, this is yet another reason why trying the Keto diet can benefit you. Everyone deals with their own stressors and tasks throughout the day, but the way that the body handles all of this can differ greatly. Your food is your fuel, so it makes sense that what you put into your body is super important for making it through each day. Most of us tend to feel completely drained by the end of a long day, but this doesn't have to be your standard way of feeling. When you put the right fuel into your body, it will actually create more energy than you've ever had before.

Keto can provide you with energy that lasts, not simply bursts that are fleeting. When you only receive energy in bursts, from coffee or sugar, for example, this creates the eventual feeling of a crash. This happens because the energy is only meant to be temporary and while it can get you through a moment, it isn't going to carry you throughout your whole day. The energy that Keto can give you is the energy that is more permanent. It is the kind of energy that builds up gradually, preventing you from ever feeling like you are going to crash.

In the Standard American Diet (SAD), carbs are overconsumed. In general, American's eat too many simple carbs, and unhealthy fats. Most of the time, the carb takes the center of the plate, with a side of protein, and little, if any, healthy fats. Additionally, we are junk food junkies - we eat too many processed foods that are often high in carbs and sugars, eat sugared "health" foods, like sugary/syrupy yogurt, and eat out at restaurants that dish out huge servings, loaded with terrible fats, a ton of carbohydrates. Because of this high intake of the wrong kind of carbs, these starches will actually be converted into glucose or sugar molecules.

Based on your knowledge of how the body works while it is not on a Keto diet, you can gather that your body is simply going to absorb the glucose and then use that for energy. This is where the fleeting energy problem becomes very real. In order to complete this process, your body needs insulin. As your glucose levels rise, so will your insulin. Even when your body has had enough, it continues to store the extra energy (glucose) for later. The insulin will also send your body signals to your liver that the glucose stores are now full. Assuming that your body is not insulin sensitive or insulin resistant, everything should go well.

As you age, though, your body can change in a way that will make it less able to handle its insulin levels properly. When your body realizes that it needs to catch up, it will demand itself to work even harder. Sometimes, it just isn't possible for it to do so. This is when you will find that many problems arise. You might find that you have unnecessary glucose in your bloodstream. If your body isn't burning it, then it simply collects until it gets the message to do something with it. During these periods, you will likely have your biggest surges of energy. However, these are the kind that can make you very tired after only a few hours later. These spurts of energy are ultimately not useful in the long run.

It is when your body's energy levels experience these drops that you begin feeling sluggish and start to crave more sugar and carbs. Since that is what you originally gave your body for this energy that you are receiving, it is naturally going to crave more of it. If you aren't careful, this can lead to unhealthy snacking and eating habits. You might find that you are craving quick snacks in order to get your fix and this usually means that you are going to reach for processed or artificial foods. You do not need to have insulin resistance in order to experience this. It is just the way that you are training your body by the diet that you are deciding to eat.

If you feel that you can identify with these energy highs and lows, you are not alone. So many people feel this way all the time, but they do not know how to tailor their diet in order to truly change the pattern. For most, adjusting the carbs that are consumed is not enough. This is when you will begin to feel hungry and cranky. Eating fewer carbs without replacing them is simply telling your body that you are giving it less fuel. This will begin an internal resistance that will likely leave you feeling frustrated. At the end of the day, you will probably still want to reach for those junk food favorites.

Keto is a way for you to ensure that you are properly replacing your carbs. When you follow a Keto diet based on the given percentages, you should be getting everything that you need in order to keep your energy levels steady. There should be no highs and lows, only medians that you will be able to reach. By receiving energy in this way, your body isn't going to think that this is the only energy it will receive for the day. Therefore, it will not go into a state of overworking followed by a big crash. Keto is all about balance and that is the one thing to keep in mind when you are seeking more energy.

Those who make the switch have expressed their concerns, much like concerns that you probably have. A lot of people worry that Keto just won't be enough to sustain them. They anticipate a lot of snacking and binge eating in order to correct this, but then they are pleasantly surprised when they realize that there is actually far less snacking needed throughout the day. When you are able to let go of the stigmas that surround the diet, you will find that your body will go through a natural process of adjustment. When you are changing anything, you need to make sure that you really commit to the change.

The Keto diet does drain all of your energy stores, but it replaces them with healthy fats. A lot of people assume that Keto is bad for you because it is like you are starving yourself, but that is not how it works. You are simply changing the way that your body operates and how it utilizes this energy. Your body isn't going to be angry with you for this switch like you might expect it to be. While it is an adjustment, your body is going to quickly realize that it can tap into the extra energy stores for more fuel whenever it needs to. It will learn what to do with these healthy fats that you are providing and how to make them last for long periods of time.

You will be able to say goodbye to your afternoon slumps and instead feel that you have enough energy to power through any day. There is also less of a chance that you will feel grumpy or "hangry" in between meals. Typically, when you are between meals, your body is waiting for you to give it more energy. Since your body stores this energy when you are on a Keto diet, there are reserves for it to dip into which truly allow you to experience your day without feeling like you are being distracted by hunger or cravings. Know that your transition into the Keto diet is going to vary. Depending on how carb-heavy your current diet is, it might take your body some time to retrain itself. For most people, it happens fairly quickly though. You might have to deal with a few days of an unsettled stomach before you truly begin to experience the benefits of Keto, but it should not be enough to deter you.

Chapter 5:
Definitive Weight Loss and
Increased Mental Clarity

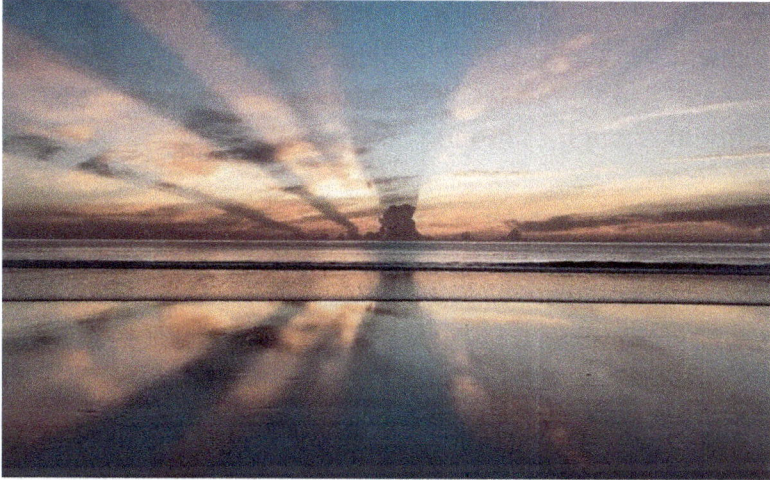

Now that you know the science behind Keto, you are likely very eager to put it to the test in your own life. With all of the benefits promised, it serves as a sustainable solution for weight management and clarity in your daily life. When your mind and body can both align, this is when you should be feeling your very best. As you begin your Keto journey, you can expect a very natural transition to take place. This is not a diet that you are going to see immediate results with, but when you start to see them, they will be long-lasting. This is not a fad diet that is going to help you shed 10lbs a week. It is a lifestyle that allows you to keep the weight off permanently. Many people who start the Keto diet have no intention of stopping and this is a healthy option if you are committed to the lifestyle.

This chapter is going to discuss what you will actually be eating while on the Keto diet. Seeing real examples of Keto-friendly menus should give you enough inspiration to create your own. When you fully understand what you should be aiming to eat, you will likely be able to think of new recipes and variations of old, familiar ones. When you are first starting out, do not have to put too much pressure on yourself to create an intricate meal plan. You can always work up to this. Having a basic and well-rounded meal plan will get you on track and it will allow you room to experiment when you feel confident enough to branch out.

Keto Ingredients

Starting out with the very basics, having knowledge about Keto-friendly ingredients is going to get you off to a good start. When you need a reminder, just think about fats and dairy. This is the basis of the diet. The following list is an example of some of the top foods that you should be reaching for while following Keto:

- Seafood (clams, muscles, oysters, squid, and octopus)
- Low-Carb Veggies (cauliflower, broccoli, and kale, leafy greens, celery, etc.)
- Cheese (especially organic, grass-fed for healthy levels of Omega 3 fatty acids)
- Avocados
- Meat and Poultry (choose grass-fed beef whenever possible, for healthy Omega 3 fatty acids)
- Eggs (choose varieties with extra Omega 3s)
- Coconut Oil (organic, extra virgin)
- Plain Greek Yogurt and Cottage Cheese (choose grass-fed for Omega 3 content)
- Olive Oil (organic, extra virgin)

- Nuts and Seeds (almonds, cashews, sunflower seeds, pecans, Macadamia nuts,
- walnuts, pistachios, pumpkin seeds, and sesame seeds)
- Berries (blueberries, raspberries, blackberries, and strawberries)
- Butter and Cream (again, preference is for grass-fed varieties for Omega 3s)
- Olives
- Unsweetened Tea and Coffee

After seeing this list of ingredients, you should be able to visualize how you can put them together in order to create nutritious meals for yourself. You can use this as a basic shopping list for your next trip to the grocery store. Shopping for your new Keto diet should not be that much different than your regular shopping trip. You have to be aware of how many carbs are in each ingredient, but otherwise, you have a lot of freedom to decide exactly what you'd like to eat for the week. For this reason, the Keto diet should never become boring or repetitive. You have so many options that you should be able to change up if necessary.

Allow yourself to explore by using some Keto-friendly ingredients in your meals that you would normally not eat on a regular basis. A handful of flax seeds in your yogurt, for example, can be a nice way to get more of your necessary nutrients without having to change the way that you would normally eat. Being crafty with these additions and substitutions will help you adjust to your new lifestyle. Eating Keto does not have to be strict and you will see just how great it will feel to be on a diet that feels like it isn't a diet. Whether you are cooking for yourself or eating outside of your home, you will be able to stick with your diet without too many issues.

Keto Food Plan

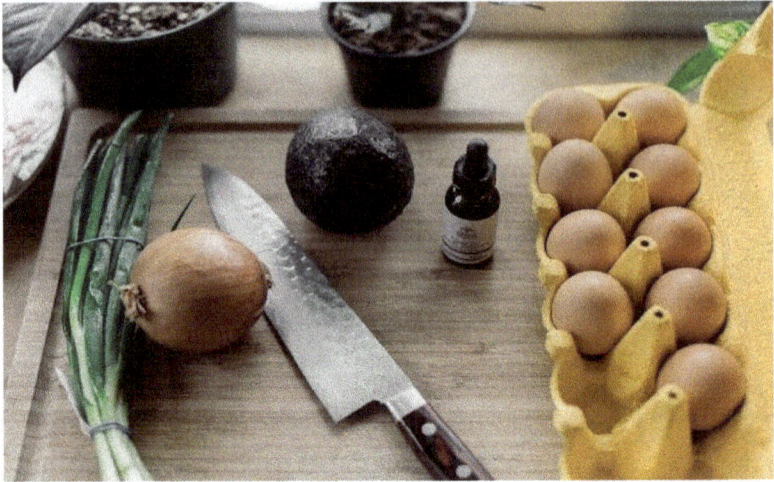

Meal planning is going to become a big part of your Keto lifestyle. When you take the time to think ahead about these things, you will feel like you are more motivated to stay on track. Deciding on what to eat when you are already really hungry is something that never goes well. When you leave it to your body to decide on this under these circumstances, this is when you are going to be most likely to give in to cravings or other unhealthy temptations that will not serve you. Meal planning is a way to keep your life organized, and while it does allow for some flexibility, it will also give you a guideline that you can continually refer to.

Breakfast, Lunch, Snacks and Dinner Meal Ideas - Week 1

1st Weekly Meal Plan

	BREAKFAST	LUNCH	SNACKS	DINNER
MONDAY	Scrambled eggs with cheddar cheese, spinach, and sundried tomatoes	Cauliflower soup with bacon or tofu	Turkey and cucumber roll-ups and celery sticks with guacamole	Garlic and herb shrimp in butter sauce with zoodles (zucchini noodles)
TUESDAY	Fried eggs with sautéed greens and pumpkin seeds	Chicken salad with cucumber, avocado, tomato, onion, and almonds	Almond milk and chia seed smoothie and berries	Beef stew with mushrooms and onions
WEDNESDAY	Omelette with mushrooms, bell peppers, and broccoli	Avocado and egg salad served in lettuce cups	Mixed nuts and sliced cheese with olives and bell peppers	Cajun chicken breast with cauliflower rice and Brussels sprouts
THURSDSAY	Almond milk smoothie containing nut butter, spinach, chia seeds, and protein powder	Shrimp and avocado salad with tomatoes, feta cheese, olives, and lemon juice	Boiled eggs and flax seed crackers and cheese	Garlic butter steak with mushrooms and asparagus
FRIDAY	2 fried eggs with avocado and a side of blackberries	Grilled salmon with leafy greens and tomato	Kale chips and sliced cheese and olives	Chicken breast with cauliflower mash and a side of green beans
SATURDAY	Egg scramble with jalapeño, green onions, tomatoes, and sunflower seeds	Tuna salad with tomatoes and avocado with a side of Macadamia nuts	Celery sticks dipped in almond butter and a handful of mixed berries and nuts	Pork chops and broccoli
SUNDAY	Yogurt and granola (low-sugar) with mixed berries	Beef burger (with no bun) with guacamole, tomato, and kale salad	Sugar-free turkey jerky and an egg and vegetable muffin	Chicken stir-fry with broccoli, mushrooms, and peppers with satay sauce

Monday:

- Breakfast — Scrambled eggs with cheddar cheese, spinach, and sundried tomatoes
- Lunch — Cauliflower soup with bacon or tofu

- Dinner — Garlic and herb shrimp in butter sauce with zoodles (zucchini noodles)
- Snacks — Turkey and cucumber roll-ups and celery sticks with guacamole

Tuesday:

- Breakfast — Fried eggs with sautéed greens and pumpkin seeds
- Lunch — Chicken salad with cucumber, avocado, tomato, onion, and almonds
- Dinner — Beef stew with mushrooms and onions
- Snacks — Almond milk and chia seed smoothie and berries

Wednesday:

- Breakfast — Omelette with mushrooms, bell peppers, and broccoli
- Lunch — Avocado and egg salad served in lettuce cups
- Dinner — Cajun chicken breast with cauliflower rice and Brussels sprouts
- Snacks — Mixed nuts and sliced cheese with olives and bell peppers

Thursday:

- Breakfast — Almond milk smoothie containing nut butter, spinach, chia seeds, and protein powder
- Lunch — Shrimp and avocado salad with tomatoes, feta cheese, olives, and lemon juice
- Dinner — Garlic butter steak with mushrooms and asparagus
- Snacks — Boiled eggs and flax seed crackers and cheese

Friday:

- Breakfast — 2 fried eggs with avocado and a side of blackberries
- Lunch — Grilled salmon with leafy greens and tomato
- Dinner — Chicken breast with cauliflower mash and a side of green beans
- Snacks — Kale chips and sliced cheese and olives

Saturday:

- Breakfast — Egg scramble with jalapeño, green onions, tomatoes, and sunflower seeds
- Lunch — Tuna salad with tomatoes and avocado with a side of Macadamia nuts
- Dinner — Pork chops and broccoli
- Snacks — Celery sticks dipped in almond butter and a handful of mixed berries and nuts

Sunday:

- Breakfast — Yogurt and granola (low-sugar) with mixed berries
- Lunch — Beef burger (with no bun) with guacamole, tomato, and kale salad
- Dinner — Chicken stir-fry with broccoli, mushrooms, and peppers with satay sauce
- Snacks — Sugar-free turkey jerky and an egg and vegetable muffin

2nd Weekly Meal Plan

	BREAKFAST	LUNCH	SNACKS	DINNER
MONDAY	Scrambled eggs cooked in butter, served on top of a bed of lettuce	Spinach salad with grilled salmon	Sunflower seeds and mixed nuts	Pork chops with red cabbage slaw
TUESDAY	Coffee made with butter and coconut oil (Google 'bulletproof coffee recipes' for some fun ideas) and hard-boiled eggs	Tuna salad stuffed in tomatoes	Mixed berries and Macadamia nuts	Meatballs served on zucchini noodles, topped with cream sauce
WEDNESDAY	Cheese and veggie omelette with salsa on top	Sashimi and miso soup (takeout)	Greek yogurt topped with crushed pecans and an almond milk smoothie with greens and protein powder	Roasted chicken with asparagus and sautéed mushrooms (in butter)
THURSDSAY	Almond milk smoothie with greens and protein powder	Chicken tenders served on a bed of greens with cucumbers and goat cheese	Hard-boiled eggs and sliced cheese with sliced bell peppers	Grilled shrimp topped with lemon and served with broccoli
FRIDAY	Fried eggs with bacon and a side of leafy greens	Burger in a lettuce bun, topped with avocado and served with a side salad	Walnuts with mixed berries and celery dipped in almond butter	Baked tofu with cauliflower rice, broccoli, bell peppers, and a Thai peanut butter sauce
SATURDAY	Baked eggs served in avocado halves	Poached salmon and avocado rolls wrapped in seaweed	Kale chips and sugar-free jerky (turkey or beef)	Grilled beef kebabs with peppers and broccoli
SUNDAY	Scrambled eggs with veggies and salsa	Tuna salad made with mayo, served in avocado halves	Dried seaweed and cheese slices	Trout broiled with butter and sautéed bok choy

Monday:

- Breakfast — Scrambled eggs cooked in butter, served on top of a bed of lettuce
- Lunch — Spinach salad with grilled salmon
- Dinner — Pork chops with red cabbage slaw

- Snacks — Sunflower seeds and mixed nuts

Tuesday:

- Breakfast — Coffee made with butter and coconut oil (Google "bulletproof coffee recipes" for some fun ideas) and hard-boiled eggs
- Lunch — Tuna salad stuffed in tomatoes
- Dinner — Meatballs served on zucchini noodles, topped with cream sauce
- Snacks — Mixed berries and Macadamia nuts

Wednesday:

- Breakfast — Cheese and veggie omelette with salsa on top
- Lunch — Sashimi and miso soup (takeout)
- Dinner — Roasted chicken with asparagus and sautéed mushrooms (in butter)
- Snacks — Greek yogurt topped with crushed pecans and an almond milk smoothie with greens and protein powder

Thursday:

- Breakfast — Almond milk smoothie with greens and protein powder
- Lunch — Chicken tenders served on a bed of greens with cucumbers and goat cheese
- Dinner — Grilled shrimp topped with lemon and served with broccoli
- Snacks — Hard-boiled eggs and sliced cheese with sliced bell peppers

Friday:

- Breakfast — Fried eggs with bacon and a side of leafy greens

- Lunch — Burger in a lettuce bun, topped with avocado and served with a side salad
- Dinner — Baked tofu with cauliflower rice, broccoli, bell peppers, and a Thai peanut butter sauce
- Snacks — Walnuts with mixed berries and celery dipped in almond butter

Saturday:

- Breakfast — Baked eggs served in avocado halves
- Lunch — Poached salmon and avocado rolls wrapped in seaweed
- Dinner — Grilled beef kebabs with peppers and broccoli
- Snacks — Kale chips and sugar-free jerky (turkey or beef)

Sunday:

- Breakfast — Scrambled eggs with veggies and salsa
- Lunch — Tuna salad made with mayo, served in avocado halves
- Dinner — Trout broiled with butter and sautéed bok choy
- Snacks — Dried seaweed and cheese slices

When you take a look at these two sample Keto weeks, it is likely that you have identified a lot of meals that you already love and enjoy on a regular basis. This becomes a great benefit of Keto because you are likely going to be familiar with most of the food you will be eating. You don't need to completely change your tastes in order to maintain a Keto-friendly lifestyle. Most of the time, you will just need to add more of certain foods and meals that you already enjoy on a regular basis. These week-long samples should serve as some inspiration as to what you would like to be eating during a typical week.

Depending on how much time you have in your current schedule, you might find that you would rather prepare most of your meals at home. There is some variety in the menus in terms of where you will be getting your food from. Takeout is still a viable option if that is something that you already utilize in your normal lifestyle. A lot of people decide that Keto is a turning point, though. They often meal prep and plan well in advance in order to ensure that they are truly maintaining their diets. Though you can eat takeout and have meals at restaurants, you must be very careful regarding the ingredients that they are using. Modifications are almost always going to be necessary.

It is a good thing for you to be aware of these options because, sometimes, eating out is going to be your only option. Whether you are meeting with a friend for lunch or having a business meeting away from the office, there will be times when you need to eat with others. A lot of us worry that being on a diet automatically means that these fun times at restaurants must come to an end and be replaced with us sitting there without a plate of food. You don't have to give up eating in its entirety in order to eat Keto all the time! The easiest way to eat out while on Keto is to focus on your protein. Almost any restaurant you go to will have a dish that is protein-focused.

After you've found your protein of choice, determine what sides it comes with. Anything carb-heavy can usually be replaced by veggies or something that contains dairy. Make sure that you ask about these substitutions before completely ruling out the entree. If you explain to the server what you can and cannot eat, you are likely to get some recommendations as well. People go out to eat while on diets all the time and restaurants generally tend to be fairly accommodating. While you are on the Keto diet, don't be afraid to ask about modifications and substitutions. Your diet plan is important to you, so treat it that way.

If you'd rather rely on your own skills to make your Keto-friendly menu, think about how to make the process even more efficient for yourself. While some people enjoy cooking every single day, others don't have the time for it. Meal prepping can help you greatly. If you can devote a single day to your grocery shopping and meal prepping, then you can likely save a lot of time when it comes to how much cooking must be done. Try to plan your menus ahead of time, taking note of recipes that sound interesting and healthy. When you have these ideas in advance, you are likely going to be able to make faster decisions in the grocery store.

Use your meal prep time as a time to unwind. Even if cooking isn't your favorite thing to do, know that you are doing this because you are making an investment towards your health. Prepare and store all of the food that you will need for the week, dividing it into portion-controlled containers. Ideally, you should sort all of the food by meal type. This way, you will be able to simply grab a portion and go or heat it up when you need to eat something. Many Keto meal prep recipes can be eaten either hot or cold, which is helpful when you are at the office or anywhere else away from your home. You might find that the whole family will become interested in your newfound meal prep ways.

If you do want to get the entire family involved in meal planning, this serves as a great way to bond and work together to come up with the plan. Eating healthy can be difficult for many reasons, but when given options, it makes the process a lot easier. Show your family the recipes you've come up with and the ones that you have grown to love. Even if they are not on the Keto diet themselves, it is highly likely that they will find your meals just as delicious as you do. Keep a recipe book handy and add new recipes to it as you see them. When you are constantly keeping track of them, you will be more likely to remember them for later.

Remember that you can utilize a mix of both eating out and cooking for yourself when you are on Keto. The key is to take a look at your lifestyle and your current schedule in order to determine what is going to work best for you. Meal prepping can be a gradual process, so if you are only able to prep for a few days at a time, try it out this way. Nothing about eating should have to be an all or nothing process. The important thing is to pay attention to your body. If you notice that you don't feel as energized when you eat at restaurants, then you are likely not getting enough nutrition. The best way to truly give your body what it needs is by preparing the food yourself. When you can listen to your body, you will always know what you need next.

Important Note

If you are not careful, you can encounter what is known as the "Keto flu." This happens when you start the Keto diet without a proper transition into the meal plan. Its symptoms can feel similar to the standard flu and it happens as the body is getting used to digesting meals without carbs. These symptoms can vary between headaches, constipation, and nausea. While many people can successfully transition into the diet without feeling any of these things, you might go through a brief period of time when you must deal with these symptoms. One of the main ways to avoid the Keto flu is by staying hydrated. If you are dehydrated, your body is being depleted of essential minerals that it needs. When water isn't enough to hydrate you, try supplementing with sugar free electrolyte beverages.

Pre-existing conditions are also important to keep in mind. If you have conditions with your pancreas, liver, thyroid, or gallbladder, the Keto diet is not going to be suitable for you. It can also cause low blood pressure and deficiencies if you do not make sure that you keep yourself on a balanced diet. To avoid this, make sure that you are taking a multivitamin regularly. Also, it is important to note that you should avoid strenuous exercise when you get started with your diet. Allowing your body the time to transition into the Keto diet before overworking itself is essential.

Chapter 6:
After Diet Appetite Control

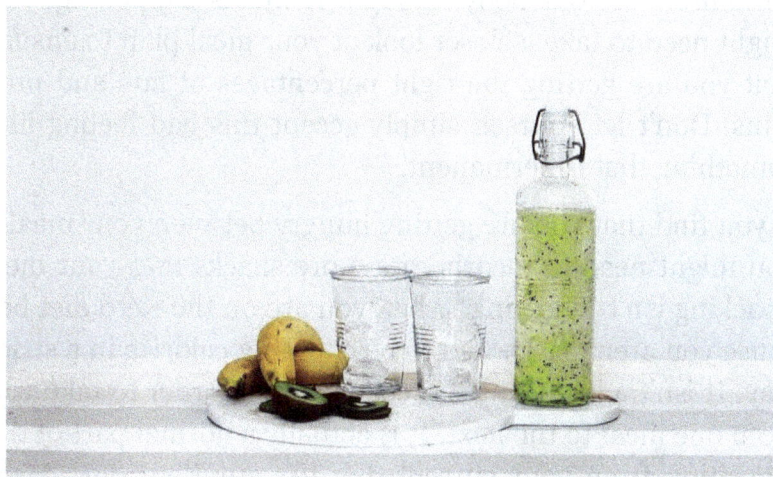

When you begin your Keto diet, an important thing to keep in mind is a method of appetite control. Any changes that are made to your normal way of eating can prompt your body to overreact and overeat. As you know, this can cause adverse effects on your body and your diet if you allow it to happen frequently. Being on any diet plan, no matter how strict or lax, requires a certain level of self-discipline. Now that you know all of the components of your Keto diet and lifestyle, you must keep them in mind at all times. When you aren't eating or snacking, your body should be in a content place. You shouldn't be craving junk food or wishing that you had more to eat. Though Keto tricks your internal systems, on a cellular level, that it is going through a period of "starvation," you should not feel this way on the outside.

Being able to recognize these red flags will ensure that you are following your Keto diet correctly. Many people wonder if it's supposed to feel bad or difficult to maintain and, in general, the answer is no. At no point should your body feel terrible compared to what it used to feel like before. Keto changes your digestive system, so some stomach pain and constipation are normal. There should not be any prolonged discomfort in your body, though. If this is happening, you might need to take a closer look at your meal plan to ensure that you are getting the right percentages of fats and proteins. Don't let yourself simply accept this bad feeling like something that is permanent.

If you find that you are getting hungry between your meals, you might need to incorporate more snacks into your diet. Snacking isn't "cheating" when you are on the Keto diet because you aren't supposed to be counting calories in a strict way. It isn't a bad thing to need snacks in order to take you from one meal to the next. It is actually a normal part of the transition from your current diet to your Keto diet. Meal prepping your snacks can be very helpful because you will always have something to reach for when you get a craving. By giving yourself only healthy and Keto-friendly snacking options, you will be less likely to stray from the path. Dividing your snacks into portion-controlled storage is also an excellent way to make sure that you are being reasonable with your cravings.

Working out might be a part of your daily lifestyle, or it might only be a part of your weekly lifestyle. No matter how often you get up and move, consider how much energy you have to burn when you do. Working out on a completely empty stomach is typically not a good idea. You will begin to feel sick or lightheaded as you get started with your workout. Try to eat something light and stay hydrated before and during your workout. After you finish up with physical activity, your body is going to need replenishment. Eating protein up to 30 minutes after a workout is going to ensure that your body has more muscle mass to build. Protein powder can also be very useful in this case, giving you a necessary boost in your smoothies before or after your workout. All you need to remember is your percentages in order to make sure that you do not overdo it with your protein intake.

Lowered Levels of Inflammation

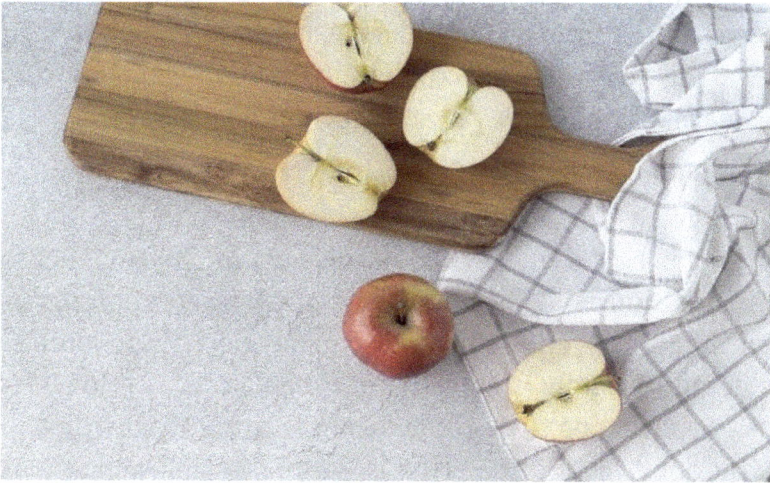

Keto is great for inflammation because it works to detoxify your body. Instead of holding on to all that sugar as it usually does, it allows your body to clean itself out. Being rid of these excess glucose stores, your body will naturally lessen the amount of inflammation that it holds onto. This is a very important benefit, especially as an aging woman because inflammation can create many problems down the road. When your joints are inflamed, many basic activities become a burden. From walking to being able to sit down in the car for longer periods of time, your body is going to be in pain if it is inflamed. Your diet has everything to do with this, as you know that the foods that are a part of the Keto plan work to combat your inflammation.

When your levels of inflammation are being properly managed by Keto, you will notice a difference when you first wake up in the morning. It is never a good idea to jump right out of bed and get moving too quickly, but that just isn't even an option when you are feeling inflamed. By getting rid of this burning and stiffness, your body will be able to adjust to being awake a lot easier. Instead of having to hit the snooze button countless times, you should be able to begin your waking up routine as soon as your alarm sounds. Get into the habit of waking up when you actually should wake up, as snoozing the alarm can create a bad start to your whole day.

Through dealing with inflammation, you have likely noticed that it gets worse when you are sitting down or standing up for long periods of time. For most of us, this means that the inflammation is at its peak while you are at work. Taking anti-inflammatory medication can be enough to dull the pain, but it usually isn't enough to keep it away for long. It is not a good feeling to be dependent on any kind of medication if you don't have to be. This is why Keto can help when it comes to an inflamed body. Instead of reaching for the medicine, you can change your eating habits to improve your inflammation. As long as you are following your Keto diet closely, it is going to begin the detoxification process right away. You should feel the impacts on your inflammation.

As you make it through your days, your body is naturally more inclined to become inflamed as you get closer to bedtime. This can prove to be very uncomfortable because you might be feeling very tired, but your inflammation is keeping you awake; maybe with restless leg syndrome, or neck and back pain. This is another point where you have likely reached for some medication in the past instead of considering what you ate for dinner. Thinking about your body as a machine that needs the right oils to operate can help you stay on track with your Keto diet. While there are always going to be temptations waiting around every corner, when you think about just how good Keto is going to make you feel, this should make it worthwhile to stick to the plan.

Inflammation is a natural part of aging. There isn't much that you can do to avoid it altogether, but preventative measures will help you in the long run. You can think of the Keto diet as a preventative approach. While it is a great diet plan, it also serves as a way to maintain your physical health by keeping you protected from these various ailments. You deserve to be on a diet that allows you to feel great *and* look great. Keto isn't simply about vanity. It allows you to get your health back on track, even if you have been unhealthy for the last several years. A common misconception is that there comes a point when it is too late to make a healthy change — it is never too late.

When you begin to live your life without your body resting in a state of inflammation, you will realize how much easier your day-to-day activities become. Starting with sleeping, you will be able to have a more restful night of sleep when your body isn't inflamed. This means that you will also be able to wake up earlier and have a more productive start to your day. Many things that you are able to accomplish happen when your body gets enough rest. If you are overworking yourself and then not making up for it with the food that you eat, you are just going to feel fatigued and down all the time.

With less inflammation also comes more potential to workout. While you don't need a bodybuilder routine, you know that getting enough physical activity into each week is an important part for any woman over 50. Staying moving will keep your body working correctly; our bodies are designed to be in motion, and not sedentary. The Keto diet will also boost your metabolism and increase your energy levels.

What you will realize is that everything in your body is connected, even if it doesn't always seem this way. Less inflammation means fewer burdens, in general. Make note of how you feel before and after your Keto diet begins. The results will likely amaze you. The best part is, there are no gimmicks in sight. Keto just works with your body.

Clean Food for a Clean Mindset

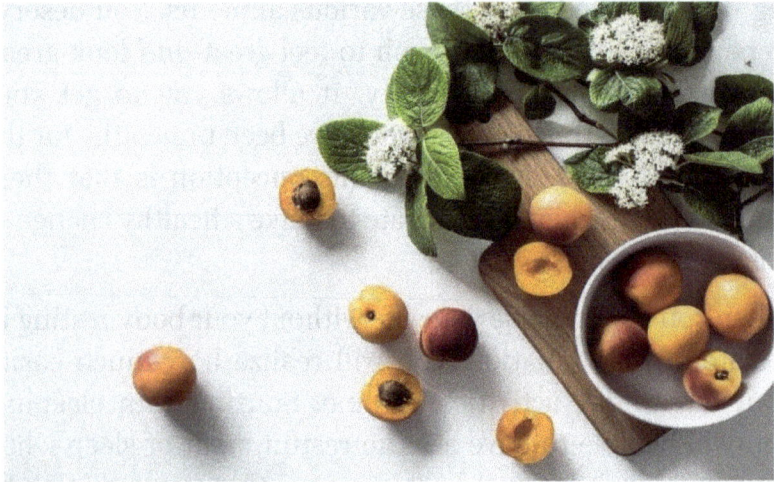

You are likely familiar with the term "clean eating," but how does that fit into your new Keto lifestyle? The principle behind eating clean is that you should aim to eat natural, whole foods whenever possible. Instead of selecting pre-packaged ingredients that contain preservatives or additives, and extra fats, sugars and salt, eating clean promotes you to only use fresh ingredients. While this can be time-consuming and difficult for those who are not used to it, eating clean will prove to be worthwhile. When your body is used to digesting real and organic food, there is less room for it to absorb any unhealthy sugars or fats. When you eat clean, you digest clean. This also allows you to have a clearer mindset.

If you aren't eating clean already, then you are likely settling yourself short when it comes to getting enough nutrients. Only natural foods have the right amount of nutrients to properly fuel your body. Even if you are eating a canned and preserved vegetable, you aren't going to be getting nearly as many nutrients as you would from eating the fresh version. It is through small changes like these that will allow you to make healthier and cleaner choices. While you don't have to opt for the organic-only grocery store, you can start by working on these smaller details.

Thinking about the foods that you are encouraged to eat while on the Keto diet, it makes sense that you are going to take a cleaner approach. In order to prepare your proteins and vegetables, it takes a simple strategy. With the occasional addition of butter or dairy, these are the ingredients that you will use to flavor the rest of the food. When you buy meat, make sure that it is always fresh. If you do have to freeze it for later, be sure to correctly label it in your freezer so it will not go bad before you get the chance to use it. Any vegetables that you will be eating on the Keto diet can be purchased fresh. It doesn't really make sense to opt for the canned versions because the fresh ones are going to taste better while providing a more nourishing benefit. If you can't get fresh vegetables, frozen veggies are a much better option than canned.

Another benefit that you can gain from eating clean comes from the knowledge that you will have access to. Being aware of what exactly is in the food that you are eating becomes an essential part of your Keto diet. When you eat clean, you will know how much protein, fat, and carbs you will be getting from eating certain foods. Not only do you need to know this information to stay on track with your Keto diet, but it also becomes helpful for you to know in general. Having an awareness of what you are eating and what it is doing to your body is very important.

Eating clean also means eating locally as much as possible. When you can utilize the ingredients in your local area, you are supporting these smaller farms as well as reducing your carbon footprint. It takes a lot of resources in order to mass-produce food which is why it makes more sense to utilize the local resources that are readily available. The planet does not have an endless supply of food, so when we can be smarter with the way that we eat, it is going to make a difference for the future. Do your best to seek out farmer's markets whenever possible. There are likely a few in your local area for you to explore. You might even discover some foods that you have never tried before because they are not typically available in regular grocery stores.

As mentioned, eating clean can also benefit your mindset. This becomes possible because of the way that eating good food can impact how you are feeling mentally. When you are eating wholesome ingredients, your body is going to respond well to this. Not only will you feel better physically, but your mental health will also see improvement. You will be able to think clearer and in a more positive way. It is almost as though your mind also goes through the same detoxification process as your body. With a clearer mind, you will see yourself doing better with various social interactions and work responsibilities. Your brain will be as sharp as it can as you navigate through all of the mental tasks that you must face each day.

If you think about it, clean eating is a savorier experience. If you were to reach for your favorite fast food burger, you would likely eat it pretty quickly. Now, imagine eating a salad with all of your favorite ingredients on it. Which one would take you longer to eat? The salad would, likely due to the fact that you have to slow down to eat it. Fast food isn't always the better option. We should not be focused on eating fast because this is actually detrimental to our physical health. When we are able to slow down the eating process and truly savor our food, we are also able to digest it better. When your body is working at a slower rate, it will know exactly how it needs to process what you are eating. Instead of eating just to simply fill yourself up, think about what your body needs. Consider what kind of fuel you can give yourself in order to be the best version of yourself possible. You'll be glad that you slowed down.

Chapter 7:
Food for Stable Blood Sugar Levels

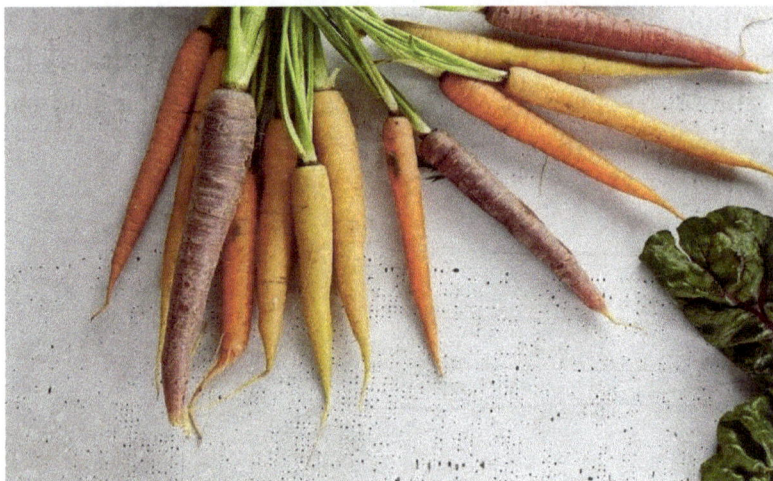

When you eat, you are likely only thinking about one thing — satisfying your hunger. While this is a big part of what eating is, it is not the only factor. The older we get, the less stable our blood sugars become. This happens naturally, and sometimes, it is to no fault of your own. The aging process isn't very forgiving unless you make an effort to manage it. If you simply allow your body to age and continue to feed it foods that do not properly nourish it, then you aren't going to be feeling the best you can feel. Eating should be a way for you to stabilize your energy levels, by keeping blood sugars in balance. It should fill you up while also replenishing your needs. If you eat junk food, you get one of these aspects. Being full is not the same thing as being healthy, though.

Consider the last meal that you ate and think about how full you got from it. Did you feel so full that you wished you hadn't eaten as much? How satisfying was the meal overall? Did you get hungry again soon after eating? These questions are all helpful tools in gauging how healthy you are with your meal choices. Even if your meals contain healthy ingredients, this does not automatically mean that you are eating in the healthiest way possible. The Keto diet helps you to reframe the way that you eat. It allows you to have large, satisfying portions while promoting clean eating simultaneously. This diet should keep you feeling healthy at all times.

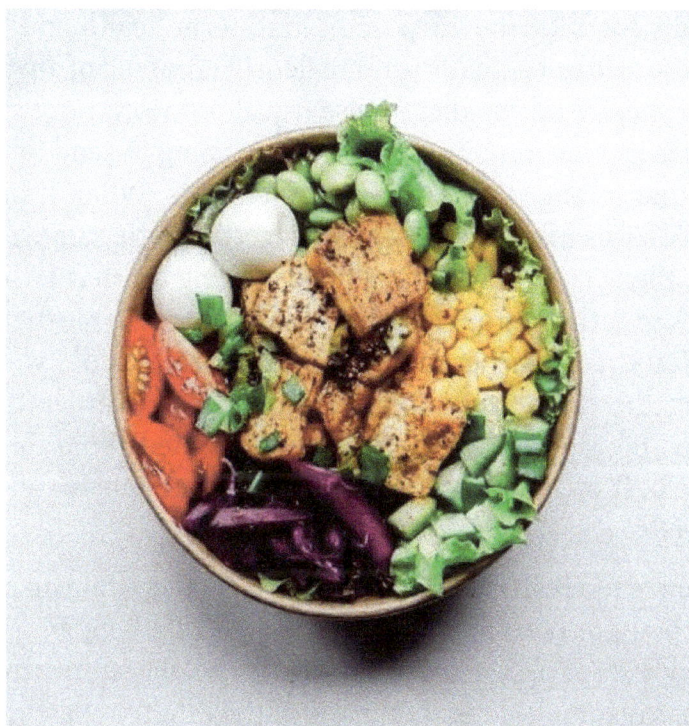

You are no stranger to the connection between carbs and blood glucose by now. When you partake in the Keto diet, you should also know how it works to eliminate this excess sugar in order to keep your body healthier. What you must keep in mind is that Keto is designed to manage your blood sugar levels, not eliminate them. We still need this glucose in order to survive. When you eat Keto-friendly foods, you are not aiming to get rid of it all in its entirety. Instead, you are aiming for a more balanced level in your body. When you have too much or too little of anything that your body makes naturally, this is going to cause you to have health problems. This is why sticking to the percentages of the Keto diet is so important. They will keep you healthy and functional, ensuring that you do not deplete your body of anything in the process.

Again, keep in mind that you are going to be eating this Keto-friendly food for the purpose of long-term health and wellness. You do not actually want to deprive yourself of anything while you are on the diet or else it will not work properly. If you are lacking anything, your body is going to send out signals that might force it to overcompensate. When it has to focus on this instead of focusing on getting into a state of ketosis, then your body is going to be missing the mark when it comes to eating Keto. This is why many people agree that eating Keto takes preparation. By reading this guide, you are taking the steps necessary that you need in order to get started the right way. When you are educated about the diet to the best of your ability, you will be better able to follow it correctly.

If you are too restrictive while on the Keto diet, this can cause your body to become insulin sensitive. This happens when the body stops producing as much glucose, therefore producing less insulin. Remember, none of the different versions of the Keto diet ask you to cut out carbs completely. While you are going to be eating a fraction of the amount that you once ate, you are still going to be getting some in your system in order to prevent these health issues. A lot of people who are unsure about the Keto diet tend to believe that the body is going to run into these problems while attempting to eat fewer carbs. Balance is everything when it comes to dieting and as long as you are following the recommended carb consumption, then you should be just fine.

On the other end of the diet, if you do not follow it closely enough, then your body isn't going to start producing and storing less glucose. This usually happens when people try to follow the diet, but do not have the willpower to keep going. This can actually be more damaging to your body than not starting Keto at all. If you are going to be doing things halfway, then you should hold off until you feel that you are ready to truly commit to the diet. You cannot expect to follow some of the rules yet get the same great results and benefits. Being realistic with your approach is going to save you from the discouragement and the hassle of not seeing the results that you are expecting.

If you ever feel that you are losing sight of your diet and what you should be eating, take a moment to regroup. Think about the benefits of the Keto diet and use them as motivation in order to keep eating properly. Cravings are natural and they will come during various points of your week. Knowing how to acknowledge them while not giving in to them will allow you to stay focused. When your blood sugar levels are changing, your body might send signals to your brain saying that it needs sugar. Know that this is just a cry for help, but that your body is going to adjust on its own in order to start burning energy from fats instead. Keep yourself calm by remembering why you are on the Keto diet in the first place and filling up on foods that are packed with healthy fats and protein instead.

Clean Food for Powerful Living

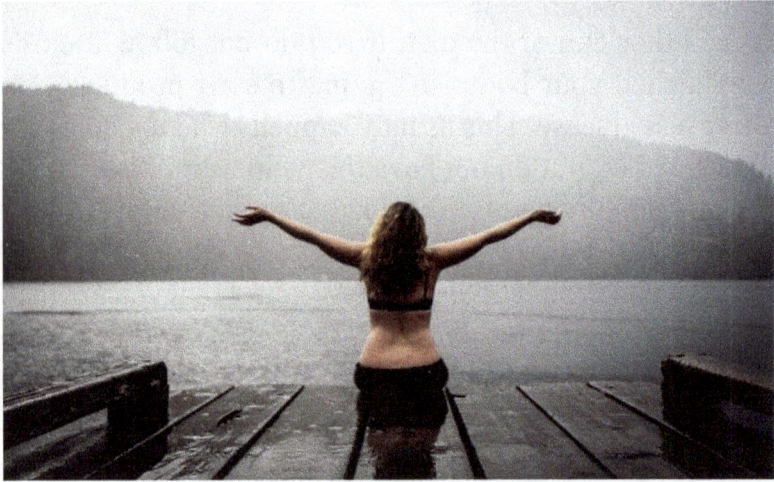

The Keto diet can definitely be thought of as a method for detoxification. In order to detox, this does not mean that you need to be empty and starving. What it means is that you are giving your body the chance to eat the purest ingredients that are free of artificial ingredients. This goes back to what we discussed earlier, with clean living, but worth a little deeper insight.

When you are choosing foods that are packaged and processed - think natural — if you can't pronounce it, then you likely don't need to be consuming it. While a lot of additives are in place to preserve the quality of the food that we eat, they are not necessarily supposed to be consumed on a regular basis. While there isn't immediate danger behind occasionally eating processed foods, your body is going to get used to them. When this happens, it makes it harder for you to switch to a clean method of eating.

Without the presence of additives, your body can take everything that you eat and turn it into something useful. Instead of having to sort through what is nourishment and what is filler, and what needs to be filtered or cleaned by your liver, your body is going to be able to go straight into the process of converting fats into energy. It will have a purpose that is clear and guided. The Keto diet aims to help provide your body with this necessary clarity. Because it does not include any ingredients that are unnecessary for your consumption, you can rest assured knowing that everything you eat is going to have its own purpose and intended use. Your body will automatically know what to do when you give it these natural ingredients to work with.

Research suggests that everyone can benefit from a detox in their diet. Even if it isn't going to be a permanent change, devoting a week or two via clean eating can do a lot in order to reset your system. The great thing about the Keto diet is that it gives you a chance to feel the benefits of a detox without having to commit to many restrictions. Most people think about going on juice cleanses when they hear the word detox, but this isn't the only way to make it happen. Just like anything else, there are levels to the process. You can detox your body while still eating just as much, if not more, food that you are used to eating.

The cravings that you will experience while you are on the Keto diet are going to challenge you. There is no way to avoid them completely, but you can be sure to build up your tolerance toward them the more you work at it. Believe it or not, the cravings do subside over time. When your body is able to detox all of the sugar from your system, it will forget what it feels like to crave it. While you will have to deal with a short period of cravings, your body is eventually going to begin craving other things. You might notice a shift in craving sugar to craving protein instead. Many people never end up trying the Keto diet because they believe that their bodies are simply going to crave sugar the whole time. If you can work your way through these initial cravings, you will find that it is actually a lot easier than you think to keep these cravings managed.

It is simply a matter of changing bad habits to good habits and shifting your mindset from the negative to the positive. This is a natural transition whenever we are changing our lifestyle, and in some ways, we're hard-wired to resist change. So, let's take a look at some ways to tackle this very common issue.

Chapter 8:
Changing Your Habits and Your Mindset to Change Your Body

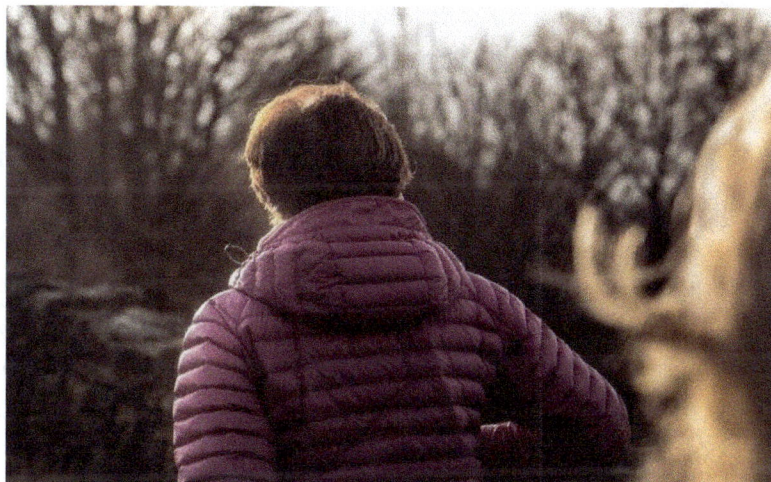

Being on a diet means following guidelines. When you already have guidelines in place, it becomes a process to switch between your current one and your new one. Try not to think about your Keto diet as a lifestyle change that is going to limit you. If you are able to see it as something that is a healthy and positive change, you are going to have a better mindset while beginning the diet. By having a clear understanding of what you should be eating and how you should be feeling, you can compare the way that you feel to the way that the diet is supposed to make you feel. This allows you to stay in control of your diet without feeling that you have to completely surrender all of your decision-making.

We all have our own bad habits, and a lot of us have bad eating habits. In today's society, it becomes easy to fall into these habits because of the promise of convenience. If you had the choice to get takeout or make a meal for yourself in a hurry, you would likely opt for takeout because you have been trained to believe that it is faster and easier. While it might be faster, you are likely compromising the quality of the food that you are eating because it appears more convenient. Most of the time, it doesn't take that much additional effort to cook for yourself. With the way that society pushes fast food and various food delivery services, it is no wonder that you would be more comfortable with allowing someone else to make your food.

While some of these services can be incredibly convenient, you are settling yourself short because you do not know exactly what you are eating. You do not know where the ingredients are from and how they were prepared. These things matter to your overall health, especially as aging becomes a factor. More than ever, you need to be paying attention to the source of your food. When you let these decisions go out of your control, you are allowing others to decide what is best for your body. Even when you begin to feel sluggish and less functional, the body becomes easily addicted to junk food so it will trick you into thinking that you need to keep eating this way.

This chapter puts focus on the things that you are already doing and how you can change them for your own health. It is hard to change your habits, but it is not impossible. As long as you have the motivation and the drive to keep moving forward, then you should be able to see real results. It often takes years to form a bad habit, so don't be discouraged if you don't notice a difference immediately. This part does take some time, but each time that you put effort into it, you are going to be working toward your main goal of becoming healthier. Tell yourself that you are doing this for your own benefit. Any time that things feel too difficult, try to get yourself back on track by remembering how great you feel when you are eating natural food that optimizes your health.

How to Make Changes: Step by Step

It becomes easier said than done when you are asked to change your eating habits. Even if you know exactly what your end result should look like, it can often be difficult to get from point A to point B. The trick is to break this part down into daily steps. You can't just expect yourself to adjust to these changes right away. The body and the mind both need time to process the changes in order to accept them as what is new and preferred. If you can commit to working on these habits each day, then you have already completed step one. Being committed to the cause is going to allow you to see real results. If you are only halfway interested in succeeding, you can imagine your results to look the same.

Start with Breakfast

You can start one meal at a time when you are planning on working on your eating habits. Think about how you start your day. Do you eat breakfast, or do you opt to wait until lunch comes around? If you choose not to eat breakfast, yet you are consuming a lot of snacks until lunch, this can become a detrimental habit. Even if you do eat breakfast, if you are loading up on sugars and carbs, this can also prove to have some negative results. Eating a balanced breakfast is how you are going to have a balanced day ahead. Your breakfast should be your fuel from the time you walk out the door until you are able to sit down and have your lunch. As you know, many will agree that breakfast is the most important meal of the day.

Even if you don't feel extremely hungry in the morning, try to eat something that will provide you with nutrition. A heavy breakfast isn't necessary but getting some protein in your body before you start your day will result in a noticeable difference. Keto breakfasts are great because they can vary in size. A lot of people feel minimal hunger when they first wake up and that is okay. Try to at least get into the habit of consuming a smoothie so that you have something in your stomach. After doing this for a week straight, you should notice that your energy levels are higher. You will also have more focus at the beginning of your day.

Stay Hydrated

As you make your way through each day, keep track of how much water you are drinking. No matter what diet you are on, drinking water is always going to be the best beverage option. Keto encourages you to drink as much water as possible. When you are hydrated, all of your bodily systems work a lot better. Water also gives you energy and fills you up when you start to have cravings. Although water cannot truly make you feel full, it can sustain you and make you feel great in between meals. If you are doing anything that is physically taxing, it is especially important to stay hydrated. As the body ages, it starts to need more hydration at a quicker pace. If you start feeling symptoms of the "keto flu," make sure you hydrate with electrolytes (sugar-free).

Avoid Sugary Drinks

If you choose a drink other than water, you need to pay attention to how much sugar it contains. Even natural fruit juices can be high in natural sugars. One of the main points of Keto is to avoid sugar, so you will have to be careful with your selection. This is why choosing water can be a simple fix because you never have to worry about how much sugar you are consuming. For a lot of people, getting rid of sodas and juices that are filled with high fructose corn syrup can be hard. Anything that you are used to becomes hard to give up.

You can try flavoring your water naturally if you need some motivation to drink it. Infuse your water with fruits for a nice added flavor.

Healthy Lunches

Think about what you can change during lunchtime. Something that matters a great deal, but people often fail to think about is the speed at which they consume their lunches. Many people will eat lunch at work or away from home and this usually happens on a timed break. If you are also in this situation, keep in mind that you shouldn't have to rush to eat your lunch. This is when you might accidentally overeat or eat too much of the wrong thing in an attempt to nourish your body. Meal planning can come in handy for lunchtime especially because you will already have a balanced meal without having to worry about it. If you don't already, consider bringing a pre-packed lunch to work.

Keto Outside the Home

You are bound to have at least a few meals outside of your home and this is definitely possible with the Keto diet, as you know. The same exact rules are going to apply, so it is up to you to request changes when necessary. If something comes with a side of carbs, ask if you can make substitutions. In many cases, you can mention that you are on the Keto diet and people will likely understand what it is that you can and cannot eat. However, when you are trying to follow any diet plan, it is your responsibility to correctly inform others who are going to be preparing your food. By explaining that you can only eat fats and dairy, there should be minimal confusion about how you need to avoid carbs.

Don't be afraid to speak up when you are eating outside of your home. This is the number one way that diets get ruined because it seems like an inconvenience to make changes. If you are truly going to commit to Keto, you need to make sure that you are monitoring your own diet. No one else is going to do this for you, which makes it even more of a victory when you can keep it up without breaking the guidelines. While Keto isn't a strict diet, you do need to be firm with yourself when you go out to eat. Sometimes, being in the presence of friends or loved ones can be tempting. If they are all eating something that you wish you could be eating, it becomes easier for you to convince yourself that you can have it too. Remember, one slip-up can mean that your body isn't going to enter ketosis. This means that the Keto diet will no longer be working the way it should.

This isn't to say that eating with others is a bad thing. Yes, you are going to have to deal with temptations, but you can still enjoy a group eating experience while still sticking to your Keto diet. When you explain to your loved ones what the diet consists of and why, they are likely going to be more sensitive to the things that you are trying to avoid. When you aren't being offered carbs and sugars, you have a higher chance of being able to forget about them and will not end up craving them as frequently. Eating around others can boost your morale because it shows you the most enjoyable parts of the experience. When you can focus on the social aspect of eating, you will end up enjoying it a lot more than if you were to focus on what you *can't* have.

Time Meals Strategically

Understand that you need time to digest your dinner. A meal that is typically eaten at home, you need to make sure that you aren't eating too close to bedtime. Since Keto does consist of a lot of meat-eating, this can feel very heavy if you are eating too late at night. When you pick a dinner time, try to stick with it. This will get your body used to digesting at a certain speed and it will get you into a regular routine. Getting into these routines is great on the Keto diet because they will keep you regulated. Try to focus on getting your nutrition in and then partaking in gentle activities. You should never eat right before you are about to lie in bed. This can upset your stomach and tell your body that it is done digesting when it actually isn't. As a result, you will likely experience insomnia or restlessness.

Keto Snacking

Change the way that you view snacking. If you have any negative connotations regarding eating snacks, you should know that this isn't necessary when you are on the Keto diet. Not only are there many Keto-friendly snacks that you can prepare for yourself, but snacking is also a very valid way to get you from meal to meal. As your body is transitioning the way that it utilizes energy, you might end up eating more snacks than you've ever eaten. This is okay! As long as you are keeping nourishing options available, then you should not be in danger of breaking your diet. A snack isn't going to fill you up like a meal will, but it should be able to hold you over until you are able to fully nourish yourself. If you are going to be out of your house for a while, it is advised that you bring a snack or two along. This will prevent you from buying food that is unhealthy for you.

Meal Prepping

Keep a recipe book in your kitchen. You can gather your favorite Keto-friendly meal ideas in one place. This way, if you ever have to prepare a meal on the spot or if you need meal prep ideas, you won't have to search for very long. You can always keep your eyes open for different recipes that you would like to try. Categorize your recipe book by the ones that you have tried and love to the ones that you would like to try in the future. If you wanted to, you could also categorize them by meal type or cuisine type. You can have a lot of creative freedom when it comes to the way that you do this, so experiment all you want! When you make it a habit to become more comfortable in the kitchen, you are going to notice this in the quality of the meals that you create.

Building New Habits - One Meal at a Time

All of these ideas are fairly simple, but they will encourage you to make important changes. Much like you had to make some changes to begin the Keto diet, you can continue to make changes in your daily life to improve your diet. Getting into a healthier mindset doesn't always happen right away, but the more that you practice, the easier it will become. You will be able to show yourself that you can manage your diet while you are away from home and you will be able to control your cravings when they hit. As long as you can keep a solid foundation, you will always be able to return to it when you need to. Keep yourself motivated by reminding yourself how you are getting healthy both inside and out.

Chapter 9:
Reaching Your Goal

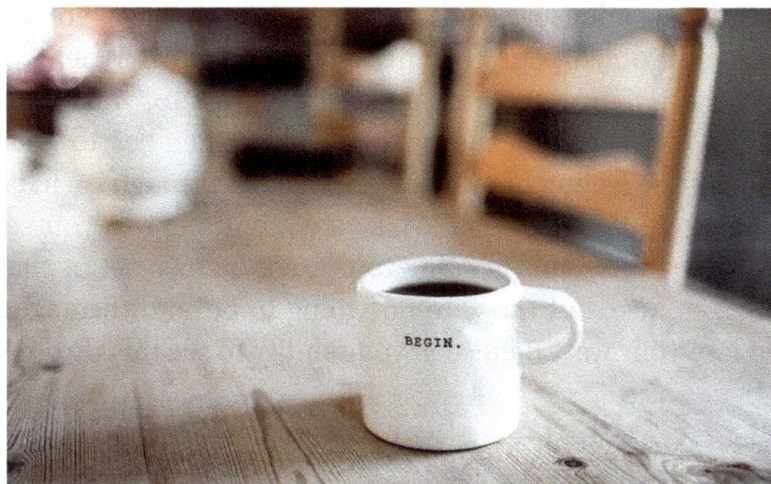

The saying remains true — you will realize that what you put into your body is going to dictate how you feel. While on the Keto diet, you are building up energy stores for your body to utilize. This means that you should be feeling a necessary boost in your energy levels and the ability to get through each moment of each day without struggling. You can say goodbye to the sluggish feeling that often accompanies other diet plans. When you are on Keto, you should only be experiencing the benefits of additional energy and unlimited potential. Your diet isn't going to always feel like a diet. After some time, you will realize that you actually enjoy eating a Keto menu very much. Because your body is going to be switching the way it metabolizes, it will also be switching what it craves. Don't be surprised if you end up craving fats and proteins as you progress on the Keto diet — this is what your body will eventually want.

Tracking Progress

Using a compare and contrast method is always great for tracking progress. Remember how you felt prior to starting the Keto diet. If you haven't started already, you can use this time to document your current state of being. Make sure to record your mindset and the cravings that you have. You can also mark down your current weight and BMI. When you have these figures to compare your progress to, you will be able to use this as a motivating tool. Remember to allow yourself the feeling of pride as you make it through each day of being on the Keto diet. Make a commitment to yourself and to the diet. This is going to present its own set of challenges to face, but they are not going to be so difficult that you lose your way. Believe in your ability to see this through.

You Are What You Eat

Think about how you used to feel while eating your sugary and carb-loaded cravings. Your immediate response is likely going to suggest that you felt great but think about the bigger picture. Did you gain more energy from eating these things? Did you experience a crash after you ate them? Instant gratification might feel great at first, but you will likely have to deal with the consequences after the fact. Eating junk food only serves your immediate cravings. It also gets your body used to craving these things by reinforcing the behavior. Junk food holds no nutritional value and it won't make you burn calories or use the sugar as a valid energy supply. When you think about it, this junk food truly doesn't have a place in your life.

Know that you can obtain happiness in other ways that don't involve eating food. While eating does tend to be a social delight, it isn't the only thing that can make you happy when it comes to food. Choose to feel happy when you can know for certain that you are treating your body properly. You should be able to feel the joy that comes from the fact that you are giving your body fuel that it can actually utilize. While eating your Keto-friendly food might not give you the same immediate rush that eating your favorite junk food does, it will benefit you much more in the long run. You will be able to notice its benefits long after you digest the food and that is what is important. A simple change in perspective is what you need to realize that your happiness isn't directly tied to the cravings that you satisfy. Your happiness needs to stem from a deeper place.

Eating tends to be an act of comfort when you are feeling down or worried. This is a cultural norm that many people experience. While being on the Keto diet, you will learn how to manage your emotions in a way that is not directly tied to the food you are eating. Instead of giving in to your cravings when you are having a hard day, the Keto diet teaches you to nourish yourself instead. When you are properly nourished, you will be able to boost your energy levels and maintain your endorphins. As you know, this will be enough to give you some extra happiness when you need it. It is a more permanent solution to your problems that tend to linger. When you can think about things from this perspective, it will be easier to remember why you are on the Keto diet at all.

No diet should make you feel so miserable that you can't even enjoy its benefits. Keto is definitely not a diet that should make you feel like you have no options. While on Keto, you should actually have the exact opposite experience. Because what you have to get rid of is so minimal, you should be equipped with many different meals that you can enjoy on a guilt-free level. Diets that torment you emotionally are not good for you, no matter how healthy you are eating. Having a healthy mind is just as important as having a healthy body. When your mindset begins to deteriorate, this will lessen your overall happiness levels. You are allowed to be happy while being on a diet! If you start to feel down, then something isn't right.

Through your example, other people will begin to see that Keto isn't as strict or difficult as they once thought. Being able to provide others with a real perspective can do a lot to keep the diet realistic. You can serve as an inspiration to your friends and loved ones with the way that you are able to stick with your diet and remain happy and fulfilled. You may have likely tried to fake this feeling while being on diets in the past, but Keto does not involve any pretending. It is important to listen to exactly how you are feeling and identify what is making you feel this way. If you begin to experience anything negative, you are encouraged to alter your diet until you begin to feel better. There should be no suffering while on the Keto diet!

Your Life Will Improve

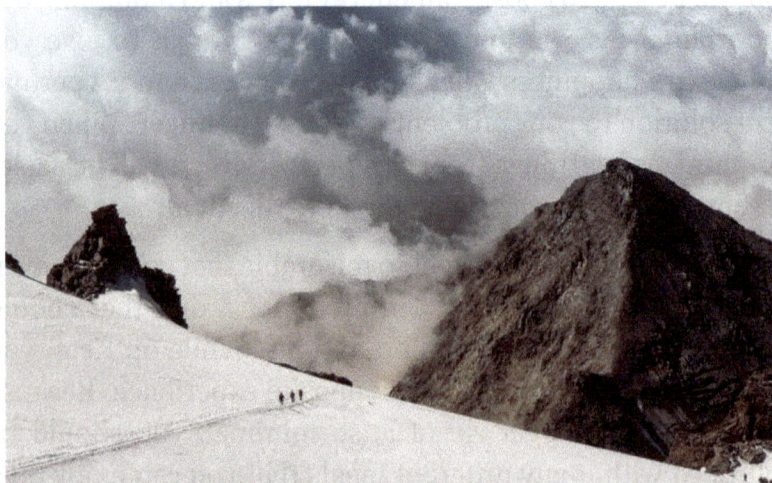

There comes a point while being on the Keto diet that you make a shift from trying to succeeding. This will happen at various points for people, but when it happens to you, embrace it. Instead of focusing on the fact that you are following a diet, you can begin to shift your focus to the benefits that you are receiving. You need to make sure that you are enjoying your life! There are so many things in life that try to get you down, so when you find something that actually brings you up, you should focus your attention on these things. One of the very first things that the Keto diet will provide you with is energy. As you have read, this is one of the benefits that you should experience fairly quickly. Use your energy to the best of your ability. Try to divide your time wisely, keeping in mind that the diet has allowed you some additional fuel to use throughout your day.

Even if you feel that your energy levels are currently on the rise, try to still practice healthy habits like going to bed earlier and waking up earlier. This is going to further regulate your bodily systems. What you need to remember is that the Keto diet is going to give you momentum. It is up to you to keep up with it. If you do nothing with it, then it is almost like these benefits are being wasted. When you can remain aware of them, you should be able to take full advantage of them. Try to practice as many healthy habits as you can when you first start noticing these new changes. This can be a very exciting and uplifting time for you!

Your Body Will Change

One of the next benefits that you will begin enjoying is the way that your appearance will change. Your skin should have a healthy glow to it, appearing youthful. As the aging process takes place, feeling ashamed of your skin can become a prominent issue that impacts your self-esteem greatly. Don't feel upset because your body is doing what it is supposed to be doing naturally. Aging is a process that no one is exempt from, but the Keto diet can help you do it more gracefully. When you notice that your skin is improving, you can make a commitment to taking better care of it. Make sure that you go to bed each night with a clean face, wear sunscreen daily, and moisturize on a regular basis. It doesn't take much to ensure that you have a solid skincare routine, so do your best to treat your skin as best as you can.

Of all the changes that Keto brings, the weight loss is probably the most anticipated. When you first begin to lose weight, you are going to feel a wave of excitement wash over you. It will become a personal challenge to keep losing weight and to keep maintaining your health. Because you are going to be burning actual fat, this weight loss isn't just a temporary experience. As long as you keep up with the Keto diet, you should be able to confidently keep the weight off with ease. Many other diets will show you quick weight loss results, but that only happens because you are losing water weight, or worse - muscle. This kind of weight tends to be a lot easier to put back on, therefore creating some discouraging results.

Whether you started the Keto diet to lose weight or to just get healthier, your body is going to begin slimming down. If you want to build muscle in the process, you need to time your workouts properly and ensure that you are getting enough physical activity each week. Knowing what forms of exercise, you enjoy will allow you to have a great workout experience. If you aren't a bodybuilder, you shouldn't have to put yourself through a bodybuilder workout routine. It just wouldn't make sense. You need to make sure that your workout plan is appropriate for your current lifestyle and experience level. You can always adjust it in the future to give yourself more of a challenge if you wish.

An often overlooked benefit to starting Keto is that you are actually going to gain a lot of experience in the kitchen. Since your meals will have to be modified, it becomes a lot easier to prepare them all yourself. While you will occasionally have meals that are prepared for you, you'll find that cooking can become a fun process. You will be learning about new food combinations and new ways to flavor the same food that you know and love. Even if you have minimal cooking experience, you should be able to create a simple Keto menu for yourself that doesn't take too much time to complete. If you work on this enough, you will start feeling more confident in the kitchen, possibly even preparing the same meals for other members of the household.

Your diet doesn't make you who you are. This is why it is possible to still enjoy every part of your life while being on Keto. The way that you eat makes up a big portion of your life, it isn't your entire life. Think about all of the other great qualities that you have that are unrelated to the Keto diet. This will make you appreciate yourself more and see that Keto is simply going to be providing you with additional benefits. You already have plenty of amazing qualities to celebrate, even without this diet. Keeping these two things separate will limit any feelings of guilt or failure when you are struggling to stay on your diet. Know that there is no diet out there that is worth destroying your self-worth over.

Having a healthy relationship with dieting is going to allow you to become your most successful version of yourself. If you start the Keto diet and end up loathing it, this isn't going to give you the best results. Your diet should be a positive addition to your life, not a burden that distresses you. Diet culture tends to teach you that you must battle with your diet in order to make it work for you. Keto is so different because there should never be this kind of a struggle. Since you are constantly listening to your body and your mind, you should only be feeling positive things.

If you are ever unsure if the Keto diet is working for you, consider all of the above factors that were discussed. Are you experiencing these benefits while still being able to enjoy your life in the way that you want to? Any time you feel limited, it is because you are unnecessarily putting these limits on yourself. Try to lighten up if you begin to feel this way. You will be able to teach yourself that it is possible to be on the Keto diet without upholding this strict sense of being. Remind yourself that you are a whole person, diet or no diet. Keto should not define you, but instead, enhance all of your great qualities. When you can realize this, you will be able to see that you are thriving. It is a fantastic feeling to know that your goals are being met and you are feeling great while doing so.

Your efforts should not only inspire those around you, but they should also serve as a way to inspire yourself. Acknowledge your progress and recognize the challenges that you had to face while arriving there. Being on a diet isn't the easiest experience at first, but you will find that you can adapt to Keto seamlessly. You will wonder what you even used to eat before. This is why Keto tends to be a permanent solution. Even those who agree to try it for a few months end up sticking with it for much longer. You should keep it up unless it no longer feels good. If you are getting all of your benefits plus the satisfaction of being full of eating clean foods, then you are likely going to continue feeling great while on Keto.

Chapter 10:
Charged with Optimism

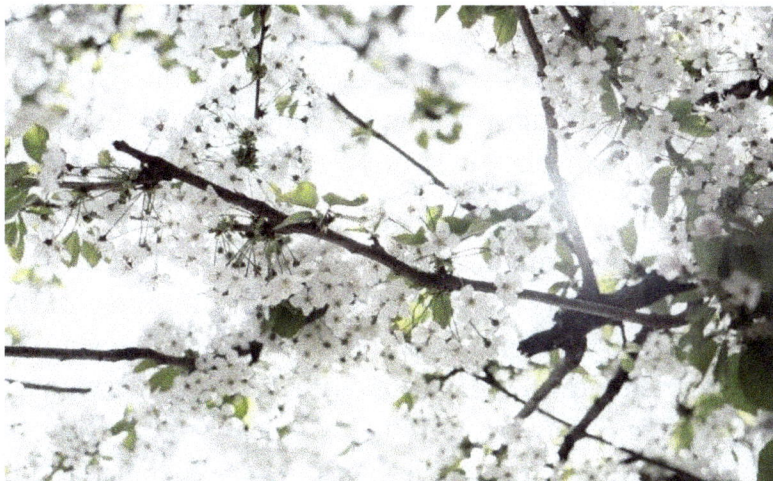

Optimism is a feeling that you will get used to while eating a Keto diet. It is a way of being that showers you with positivity in every aspect of your life. While you are going to always face challenges and setbacks in your life, having an optimistic outlook is going to help guide you through anything that you encounter. Certain things can feel discouraging the older that you get because it becomes harder to correct them. Taking care of your body and losing weight can be a couple of those things. If you no longer have hope that you can accomplish certain things, then it is not going to be easy to stay optimistic. This is how being on the Keto diet can help you. Everything that it does for your body aligns with an optimistic outlook. Because you will be taking care of your mind and body, this leaves little room for pessimism.

Before you even begin your diet, it is a wise idea to reevaluate your life. Think about what you do to cope with things when they get difficult. You might find that your coping abilities are not up to par when you realize that they revolve around eating poorly or not getting enough nutrients. Recognize these habits without putting any blame on yourself. By simply identifying them, you will have a better idea of what needs to change. When you can reevaluate yourself while keeping a neutral mindset, you will be more likely to make productive changes in your life. Acknowledge that you might not have the healthiest coping mechanisms at the moment, but this can change if you truly want it to.

Think about what you truly want for yourself and what you truly want out of your life. Try to think beyond the things that give you instant gratification. This can be a deep realization to come to, so it is important that you do not rush yourself. You can meditate on the idea or write down your thoughts in order to keep them organized. Try to only think about the things that will actually serve your purpose and allow you to meet your goals. By getting rid of the idea that temporary fixes are going to help you, then you will be able to focus on what is really most important. It can be difficult to truly dissect these things, but it is good to have an idea of where you currently are in your life. This is all going to matter as you begin your Keto journey.

Make a pact to get rid of your bad habits and bring in the new habits to take their place. When you have a solution present, it feels less like you are giving up on something and more like you are simply reframing your way of thinking. This is how you are going to keep the optimism flowing freely while you are on the Keto diet. Never take anything away from yourself, food or otherwise, without first thinking of a positive replacement for it. When you do things this way, you will never feel like you are being deprived of the things that you want the most. You will instead be teaching yourself and your body how to desire healthy alternatives.

Food and happiness are closely linked in more ways than you think. Aside from eating foods that comfort you when you are feeling down, there are actually some foods that naturally boost your happiness because they are good for your brain. These foods often fall into the protein category and they work by keeping your brain active and sharp. When you do not exercise your brain, much like any other muscle in your body, it becomes weak and tired. Doing so becomes a hassle because it feels like it is not able to function as it once used to. By eating healthy fats and omega 3 rich proteins on a daily basis, your brain is going to have the fuel to stay active. It will be exercising itself and functioning at its prime. This will keep you happier because you will be aware of exactly what you are doing and feeling.

When you do not have a clear head, life can become complicated. Living with this cloud hovering over you can often feel like something is wrong when everything is actually okay. The brain is very powerful, and it can lead you to many different conclusions if you are not careful. One major factor to look into if you begin to experience depression is your diet. While it might seem trivial, it is a factor in the way that your brain operates. You might be going through a lot of dark, personal issues but that isn't the only problem. If you fill your body with junk food and preservatives, it doesn't get the proper nutrients to produce the right chemicals in your brain that will make you happy. Instead, it will just be running off of sugar until it crashes and then the cycle repeats.

Staying optimistic while on the Keto diet does require some basic knowledge about the brain. A depressed brain is harder to keep happy if you aren't eating food that is packed with nutrients. After your first week full of protein, make note of how your brain feels and how clear your thoughts are. Most likely, you will find that you are able to think much clearer with more confidence. Being able to use your brain in the way that you know you are capable of provides you with a sense of purpose and stability. This is important to any human being because living without a purpose is one way to trigger depression. This can make life feel very overwhelming and scary. Being on Keto is great because you have an automatic purpose. When you feel the benefits of the results in your brain, this is just another positive aspect of the diet making its way into your lifestyle.

Keeping Yourself Inspired

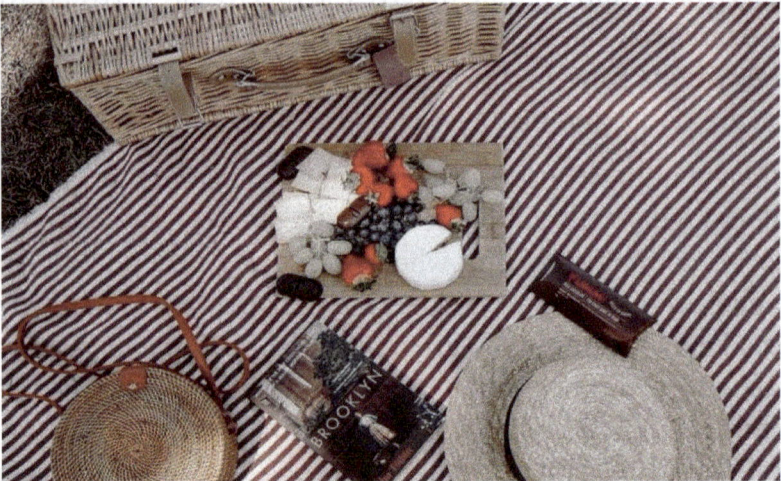

It is important to seek out inspiration with everything that you do in life. Having a source of inspiration will provide you with even more motivation to reach your goals. In a way, this guide can serve as your first source of inspiration as you begin your Keto journey. By reading about the facts and benefits of the lifestyle, you should feel excited and ready to begin. Once you get the hang of Keto, you start to become your own inspiration. You can do so by being persistent with your routine.

Everyone has routines that they follow throughout the day, whether they change frequently or remain the same. Having routines means that you have a sense of stability, which is great! Your routine should be regular enough to keep you on track, yet flexible enough to never become boring or stale. A great routine has room for mistakes and plenty of room for changes, if necessary.

Each morning recite some positive affirmations to yourself as you begin your day. These affirmations can be as simple as "I can do this," or as complex as you want them to be. No matter what is going on in your life, if you start the day with positivity, you are likely going to be able to return to this positivity later on. Use your breakfast time as a chance for you to enjoy the fact that you are nourishing your body. No matter what you are eating, any Keto breakfast is going to prepare you for the day ahead. If you are bringing lunch with you to work, make sure that it is packed and ready to go with you. Without having to struggle to decide what you'd like to eat for lunch that day, you are taking away one stressor. The more stressors that you are able to eliminate, the better your day will go.

Remember to savor your lunch once you get the chance to eat it. Sit down and enjoy your food. Let the quality and healing properties of the food inspire you. Your lunch break should be used for eating and nothing else. If you are multitasking during this time, your body isn't going to reach a state of relaxation. All of the tension and stress that you have been holding onto throughout the morning is going to follow you as you eat your lunch. This can cause your digestive system to act up, potentially even causing you indigestion or an upset stomach. Stress tends to build up in your stomach which can definitely influence your appetite. Know that no matter what is going on around you, you'll be able to return to it after you enjoy your lunch. It's amazing what a few moments of relaxation can do to break up all of the different elements that you have been experiencing throughout your day.

If you do find an opportunity to eat out with your friends, take this as a personal challenge of your knowledge about the Keto diet. Think about any substitutions that can be made to classic restaurant food. Know that you shouldn't be ashamed that you are focused on your health. Being on a diet isn't the end of your fun and happiness. It is meant to become a regular part of your lifestyle. Your friends and loved ones should also be understanding and supportive of your cause. If you show them how the Keto diet is making you feel great, then there is no reason why the ones who care about you most would make you feel guilty for being on the diet. Your support system is very important during this time, so make sure that you are aware of the company that you are keeping. A good support system should be an inspirational, encouraging and supportive voice while you are on your journey. You might even find that they will become interested in trying out the diet for themselves.

As you have been learning about the Keto diet for yourself, it is likely that you have been able to see past many of the stigmas that people talk about. This happens with nearly any diet plan because dieting has been a controversial topic in society for the last several decades. By spreading accurate information about the Keto diet and being a living example of someone who is on it, you are doing your best to educate those around you. When you can show people that you aren't actually "starving" and that you are receiving benefits such as weight loss and energy boosts, this can truly change minds about how the Keto diet really works. People are going to be naturally skeptical, but as long as you stay true to what you know, you will be able to continue seeing the successful results that you desire.

Let dinner time be your chance to explore new options. Whether you are eating in with the family or going out to a new restaurant, try to have something new for dinner each night to keep you intrigued with the diet. There are so many options for what you can make given the ingredients that Keto boosts. You will always have a protein-packed entree that is full of flavor. Because you are able to cook with butter and oil, all of your favorite dishes can be replicated without having to skip over them. People truly enjoy how many of their favorite savory meals are included in the guidelines of the Keto diet. Some people say that it almost feels too good to be true that they are still able to eat these things! Eating healthy, healing foods is definitely a source of inspiration.

When you take the time to make sure that your body feels great by exercising, know that this is a reason to be inspired by yourself and your choices. It can be difficult to get up and moving, especially while on a new diet. Commend yourself for the effort that you put into your workout routines and know that, paired with the Keto diet, you are going to be seeing results very soon. When you get into these habits, you will be more likely to return to them again in the future on your own. They become less like tasks to complete and more like normal parts of your day that you can expect. When you get into the full swing of Keto, it should feel natural and effortless.

Conclusion

Now that you are familiar with the Keto diet on many levels, you should feel confident in your ability to start your own Keto journey. This diet plan isn't going to hinder you or limit you, so do your best to keep this in mind as you begin changing your lifestyle and adjusting your eating habits. Packed with good fats and plenty of protein, your body is going to go through a transformation as it works to see these things as energy. Before you know it, your body will have an automatically accessible reserve that you can utilize at any time. Whether you need a boost of energy first thing in the morning or a second wind to keep you going throughout the day, this will already be inside of you.

As you take care of yourself through the next few years, you can feel great knowing that the Keto diet aligns with the anti-aging lifestyle that you seek. Not only does it keep you looking great and feeling younger, but it also acts as a preventative barrier from various ailments and conditions. The body tends to weaken as you age, but Keto helps to keep a shield up in front of it by giving you plenty of opportunities to burn energy and create muscle mass. Instead of taking the things that you need in order to feel great, Keto only takes what you have in abundance. This is how you will always end up feeling your best each day.

Arguably one of the best diets around, Keto keeps you feeling so great because you have many meal options! There is no shortage of delicious and filling meals that you can eat while you are on any of the Keto diet plans. You can even take this diet with you as you eat out at restaurants and at friends' houses. As long as you can remember the simple guidelines, you should have no problems staying on track with Keto.

Cravings become almost non-existent as your body works to change the way it digests. Instead of relying on glucose in your bloodstream, your body switches focus. It begins using fat as soon as you reach the state of ketosis that you are aiming for. The best part is, you do not have to do anything other than eating within your fat/protein/carb percentages. Your body will do the rest on its own.

Because this is a way that your body can properly function for long periods of time, Keto is proven to be more than a simple fad diet. Originating with a medical background for helping epilepsy patients, the Keto diet has been tried and tested for decades. Many successful studies align with the knowledge that Keto really works. Whether you are trying to be on the diet for a month or a year, both are just as healthy for you. Keto is an adjustment, but it is one that will continue benefiting you for as long as you are able to keep it up. If you are ready to feel great and look great from the inside out, you can begin your Keto journey with the confidence that it is truly going to make a difference in your life. The natural signs of aging and hormonal imbalances of being a woman are not enough to hold you back when you are actively participating in a balanced Keto diet.

Change your life today and enjoy the many benefits of a Keto diet.

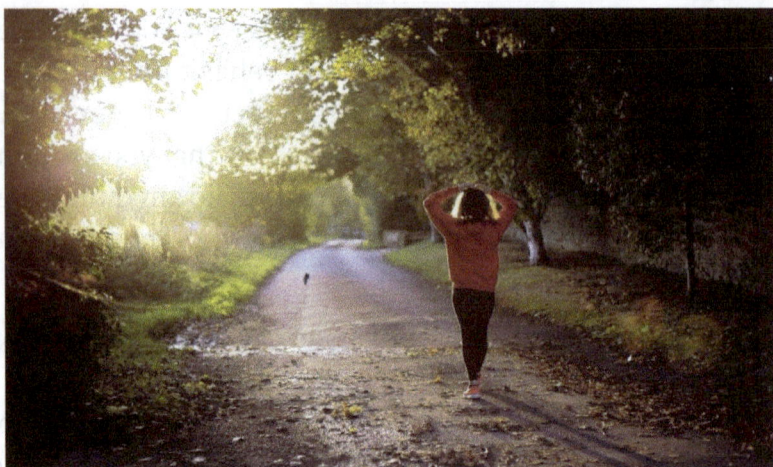

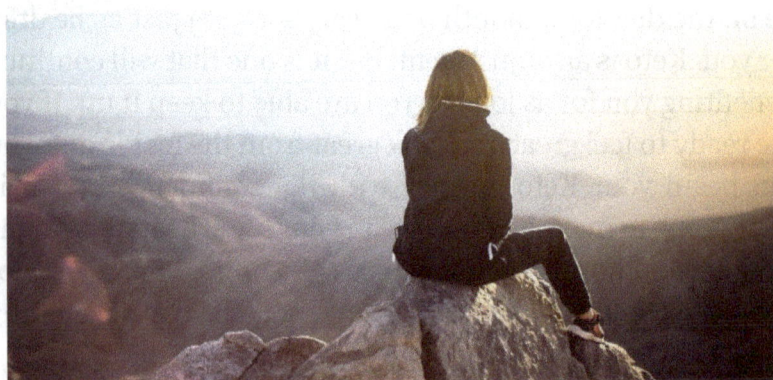

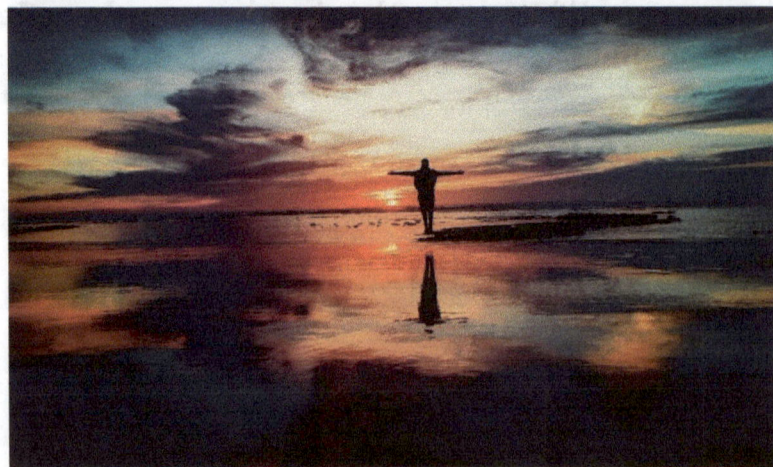

References

Alley Interactive. (2020, January 6). This Anti-Aging Keto Plan Helps You Shed Pounds in a Flash. Retrieved February 4, 2020, from https://www.wom-answsworld.com/posts/diets/anti-aging-keto-172222

Ciccarelli, D. (2019, September 13). Keto Energy: How a Ke-togenic Diet is the Secret to Sustained Energy. Re-trieved February 4, 2020, from https://perfect-keto.com/keto-energy/

Ciccarelli, L. (2019, November 26). Keto For Women: How to Do It Right and Lose Weight. Retrieved February 4, 2020, from https://perfectketo.com/keto-for-women/

Clarke, C. (2019, September 13). Targeted Ketogenic Diet: An In-depth Look. Retrieved February 4, 2020, from https://www.ruled.me/targeted-ketogenic-diet-in-depth-look/

Dunn, S. T. (2019, June 3). 10 Reasons to Eat Clean. Re-trieved February 4, 2020, from https://www.cleaneatingmag.com/clean-diet/10-reasons-to-eat-clean

Healthy Eating: Changing Your Eating Habits. (2020). Re-trieved February 4, 2020, from https://wa.kaiser-permanente.org/kbase/topic.jhtml?docId=ad1169

Hyman, M., MD. (2019, October 21). 7 Reasons You Need to Detox! Retrieved February 4, 2020, from https://drhyman.com/blog/2015/03/12/7-reasons-you-need-to-detox/ Kubala, M. (2018, April 3). The

Keto Flu: Symptoms and How to Get Rid of It. Retrieved February 10, 2020, from https://www.healthline.com/nutrition/keto-flu-symptoms#get-rid

Kubala, M. J. S. (2018, October 30). What Is the Cyclical Ketogenic Diet? Everything You Need to Know. Retrieved February 4, 2020, from https://www.healthline.com/nutrition/cyclical-ketogenic-diet#basic-steps

Leonard, J. (2020, January 29). Keto diet: 1-week meal plan and tips. Retrieved February 4, 2020, from https://www.medicalnewstoday.com/articles/327309.php#1-week-sample-meal-plan

Mawer, R. M. (2018, July 30). The Ketogenic Diet: A Detailed Beginner's Guide to Keto. Retrieved February 4, 2020, from https://www.healthline.com/nutrition/ketogenic-diet-101#types

Migala, J. (2019, November 4). The Keto Diet: 7-Day Menu and Comprehensive Food List | Everyday Health. Retrieved February 4, 2020, from https://www.everydayhealth.com/diet-nutrition/ketogenic-diet/comprehensive-ketogenic-diet-food-list-follow/mindbodygreen. (2019, October 24).

Why The Ketogenic Diet Is Great For Hormone Balance. Retrieved February 4, 2020, from https://www.mindbodygreen.com/articles/why-the-ketogenic-diet-is-great-for-hormone-balance

Occhipinti, M., PhD. (2018, September 10). What is the History and Evolution of the Keto Diet? Retrieved February 4, 2020, from https://www.afpafitness.com/blog/what-is-the-history-and-evolution-of-the-keto-diet

Spritzler, R. F. D. (2017, January 23). 16 Foods to Eat on a Ketogenic Diet. Retrieved February 4, 2020, from https://www.healthline.com/nutrition/ketogenic-diet-foods#section1

StockSnap.io - Beautiful Free Stock Photos (CC0). (2020c). Retrieved February 4, 2020, from https://stocksnap.io/

www.ingramcontent.com/pod-product-compliance
Lightning Source LLC
Chambersburg PA
CBHW060312030426
42336CB00011B/1014